Manual of
URODYNAMICS

Manual of URODYNAMICS

Mayank Mohan Agarwal
MBBS MS (Surg) DNB (Surg) MRCS (Ed) MCh (Urol) DNB (Urol)
Assistant Professor of Urology
Postgraduate Institute of Medical Education and Research
Chandigarh, India
Urology Specialist
New Medical Center Specialty Hospital
Abu Dhabi, UAE

Foreword
Gopal Badlani

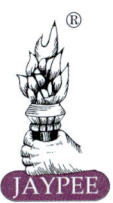

JAYPEE BROTHERS MEDICAL PUBLISHERS (P) LTD
New Delhi • London • Philadelphia • Panama

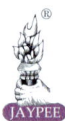

Jaypee Brothers Medical Publishers (P) Ltd

Headquarters

Jaypee Brothers Medical Publishers (P) Ltd
4838/24, Ansari Road, Daryaganj
New Delhi 110 002, India
Phone: +91-11-43574357
Fax: +91-11-43574314
Email: jaypee@jaypeebrothers.com

Overseas Offices

J.P. Medical Ltd
83 Victoria Street, London
SW1H 0HW (UK)
Phone: +44-2031708910
Fax: +02-03-0086180
Email: info@jpmedpub.com

Jaypee Medical Inc
The Bourse
111 South Independence Mall East
Suite 835, Philadelphia, PA 19106, USA
Phone: +1 267-519-9789
Email: jpmed.us@gmail.com

Jaypee Brothers Medical Publishers (P) Ltd
Bhotahity, Kathmandu, Nepal
Phone: +977-9741283608
Email: kathmandu@jaypeebrothers.com

Jaypee-Highlights Medical Publishers Inc
City of Knowledge, Bld. 237, Clayton
Panama City, Panama
Phone: +1 507-301-0496
Fax: +1 507-301-0499
Email: cservice@jphmedical.com

Jaypee Brothers Medical Publishers (P) Ltd
17/1-B Babar Road, Block-B, Shaymali
Mohammadpur, Dhaka-1207
Bangladesh
Mobile: +08801912003485
Email: jaypeedhaka@gmail.com

Website: www.jaypeebrothers.com
Website: www.jaypeedigital.com

© 2014, Jaypee Brothers Medical Publishers

The views and opinions expressed in this book are solely those of the original contributor(s)/author(s) and do not necessarily represent those of editor(s) of the book.

All rights reserved. No part of this publication may be reproduced, stored or transmitted in any form or by any means, electronic, mechanical, photocopying, recording or otherwise, without the prior permission in writing of the publishers.

All brand names and product names used in this book are trade names, service marks, trademarks or registered trademarks of their respective owners. The publisher is not associated with any product or vendor mentioned in this book.

Medical knowledge and practice change constantly. This book is designed to provide accurate, authoritative information about the subject matter in question. However, readers are advised to check the most current information available on procedures included and check information from the manufacturer of each product to be administered, to verify the recommended dose, formula, method and duration of administration, adverse effects and contraindications. It is the responsibility of the practitioner to take all appropriate safety precautions. Neither the publisher nor the author(s)/editor(s) assume any liability for any injury and/ or damage to persons or property arising from or related to use of material in this book.

This book is sold on the understanding that the publisher is not engaged in providing professional medical services. If such advice or services are required, the services of a competent medical professional should be sought.

Every effort has been made where necessary to contact holders of copyright to obtain permission to reproduce copyright material. If any have been inadvertently overlooked, the publisher will be pleased to make the necessary arrangements at the first opportunity.

Inquiries for bulk sales may be solicited at: jaypee@jaypeebrothers.com

Manual of Urodynamics

First Edition: **2014**

ISBN: 978-93-5152-187-7

Printed at: Samrat Offset Pvt. Ltd.

Dedicated to

Dear readers and the patients

Foreword

Tell me and I forget. Teach me and I remember. Involve me and I learn.
—Benjamin Franklin

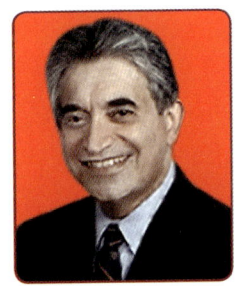

It is my pleasure to write this Foreword for Dr Mayank Mohan Agarwal's new book on Manual of Urodynamics.

To me, Urodynamics (UDS) is a study which explains the pathophysiology of many lower urinary tract symptoms and some upper urinary tract ailments. Many make it into a voodoo science and complicate it enough that most students and residents run away from it.

This manual is intended for all the students and practitioners of urology, urogynecology and gynecology, who are interested in UDS. It is well-illustrated and explains various topics related to urology in an easy-to-understand language. It is full of clinical examples with illustrative cases. The reader will be able to walk the path from initial assessment with a bladder diary to complex multichannel VUDS with the help of this manual. It also clarifies several obscure urodynamic theories and introduces novel and useful concepts (e.g. volume-normalized flow-rate index and micturitional UPP). Emphasis has been laid on making an individualized choice of different urodynamic studies using appropriate examples. He has tried to describe some difficult concepts (e.g. Schafer nomogram DAMPF) in simple language.

I have had the privilege of watching Dr Agarwal first-hand and interacted with him at numerous conferences. He has an indepth knowledge of the subject but, most importantly, he has the desire to teach and share his knowledge with many. He does so by involving the learners in the learning process rather than talk to them.

This concise book should be a handy guide for many.

Gopal Badlani MD
Professor of Urology and Vice Chair of Clinical Affairs
Department of Urology
Wake Forest Baptist Medical Center
Winston Salem, NC, USA

Secretary General
American Urological Association
Baltimore, MD

Preface

"You must read, you must persevere, you must sit up nights, you must inquire, and exert the utmost power of your mind. If one way does not lead to the desired meaning, take another; if obstacles arise, then still another; until, if your strength holds out, you will find that clear which at first looked dark."
—Giovanni Boccaccio

Understanding of urodynamics (UDS), literally a study of dynamics of collection and voiding of urine in lower urinary tract, is essential for any urologist treating patients with lower urinary tract symptoms. It cannot be overemphasized that the term 'urodynamics' encompasses simple noninvasive tests, i.e. bladder-diary, uroflowmetry as much as the complex invasive studies, i.e. video urodynamics, electromyography.

UDS has long borne a tag of being impractical/too difficult for 'routine clinical practice' by most urologists and, therefore, not used optimally. Moreover, there has been confusion prevailing amongst the practitioners of the craft regarding the indications of and definitions used in various urodynamic studies. The lack of interest of urologists in this marvelous 'art' is not entirely ill found, since there actually is a large gray area concerning indications, performance, definition and interpretation of various aspects. Over the years of my training and practice, through studies, research, interactions with experts in the field and keen observations of patients' clinical picture, I, along with my colleagues, have been able to unfold several obscurities. While writing this *Manual of Urodynamics*, I have kept the following goals in mind:

- Simple understanding for performance of each urodynamic test
- Troubleshooting of difficulties encountered during the test
- Interpretation of individual results—basic as well as advanced
- Conceptualization of individualized indications of each test
- Clarification of obscure areas through personal experience and research data.

To accomplish the goals and for interesting reading, the whole book has been made full of graphs, images, explanations and examples. There is a full chapter on representative clinical cases, in which I have shown how the clinical query was generated and how the appropriately performed UDS could help make clinical decisions.

Urodynamics is an interesting and illustrative science with a lot of scope for discussion. The expected readership of this manual is students, practitioners as well as researchers of Urology, Urogynecology and Gynecology at all stages of their career, if they have an inclination of proper management of patients with lower urinary tract symptoms. After reading this book, several concepts will be clarified. Nevertheless, new queries will be generated. It will be my utmost pleasure to respond to any queries, comments, complaints and suggestions of my dear readers.

Mayank Mohan Agarwal

Acknowledgments

I am deeply indebted to my respected teachers Dr AK Mandal and Dr SK Singh for creating an environment conducive to interactive learning, encouragement and development in our department. My colleague Dr Ravimohan has always been there for discussion, constructive criticism and suggestions in every aspect of my professional life, and writing of this book being no exception. I can never thank enough my residents, the pillars for years of my clinical and research work in the field of urodynamics. I'd particularly like to thank Dr Yogesh, Dr Saurabh, Dr Manish, Dr Sathish, Dr Sudheer, Dr Sunirmal, Dr Mayur, Dr Shiva, Dr Kishore, Dr Krishna Kishore and Dr Ranjan.

My lovely wife Dr Niti and children Aryan and Atharv are my ultimate source of inspiration and encouragement in whatever I do, including this work. I cannot describe gratitude towards my and my wife's parents in words for being always there and for their unspoken appreciation and encouragement.

Lastly, I am grateful to my patients, who helped me understand the intricacies of lower urinary tract function, through keen interaction with them and through ethical research.

Thank You God!

Contents

1. **Anatomy and Physiology of the Lower Urinary Tract**   1
   - Anatomy of the Lower Urinary Tract   1
   - Function of the Lower Urinary Tract   3
   - Neural Control of the Lower Urinary Tract   4

2. **Clinical Assessment of a Patient with Lower Urinary Tract Symptoms**   7
   - History   7
   - Examination   8

3. **Uroflowmetry**   13
   - Types of Uroflowmeters   14
   - Standardization Requirements of the Equipment   15
   - How to Read and Interpret Uroflow Data   16

4. **Cystometry and Pressure-flow Study**   23
   - Hardware   23
   - The Filling Phase   33
   - The Micturition Phase   38

5. **Video Urodynamics**   49
   - Setup   49
   - Procedure   51
   - Indications of Video Urodynamics   51
   - Advantages of VUDS (or VCUG Done Separately within a Short Interval)   54

6. **Urethral Pressure Profilometry (UPP)**   58
   - Stress UPP   63
   - Micturitional UPP (MUPP)   65

7. **Ambulatory UDS**   71
   - Technique   72
   - Interpretation   73

8. **Whitaker Test**   75
   - Procedure   75
   - Interpretation of Results   76
   - Role of Whitaker Test   76
   - Drawbacks of Whitaker Test   77

9. Representative Case Discussion 79
- Patient 1 79
- Patient 2 81
- Patient 3 85
- Patient 4 86

10. Reporting Urodynamics 89
- Filling Phase 89
- Stress Phase 90
- Micturitional Phase 91

Index 93

Abbreviations

AG	Abrams-Griffiths number
BOOI	Bladder outlet obstruction index
cQave	Volume-Corrected Qave
cQmax	Volume-Corrected Qmax
DAMPF	Detrusor adjusted mean passive urethral resistance relation factor
DCI	Detrusor contractility index
DOI	Detrusor overactivity index
LUT	Lower urinary tract
LUTS	Lower urinary tract symptoms
MCC	Maximum cystometric capacity
MUCP	Maximum urethral closure pressure
OCO	Obstruction coefficient
Pabd	Abdominal pressure
Pclo	Urethral closure pressure
Pdet	Detrusor pressure
Pura	Urethral pressure
Pves	Vesical pressure
PVR	Postvoid residual urine
Qave	Average flow rate
Qmax	Maximum flow rate
UDS	Urodynamic study
UPP	Urethral pressure profilometry
VE	Voiding efficiency
VUDS	Video-urodynamic study
VV	Voided volume

CHAPTER 1

Anatomy and Physiology of the Lower Urinary Tract

A detailed description of complete anatomy and physiology of lower urinary tract is vast and beyond the scope of this book. Nevertheless, a brief mention of the same pertaining to functional understanding of the tract would be relevant here and is described as under.

ANATOMY OF THE LOWER URINARY TRACT

Bladder is divided into two parts—body and base. The base comprises of trigone and bladder neck. The bladder base and posterior urethra along with its muscular surroundings (prostate and sphincteric muscles) are collectively known as 'the bladder outlet'. In males, the posterior urethra (or the flow-controlling zone) comprises of pre-prostatic, prostatic and membranous parts which then continues as bulbar urethra beyond the pelvic floor musculature. In females, the urethra is short and almost the whole of it is the flow-controlling zone. It is often divided into proximal, mid and distal urethra.

On luminal aspect, the bladder is lined by 6-cell-layered transitional epithelium resting on a basement membrane. The epithelial unit rests on fibromuscular lamina propria, which allows considerable distension. The muscular architecture of bladder is appropriate for emptying of a spherical structure. The smooth muscle is roughly arranged into inner longitudinal, middle circular and outer longitudinal layers. The muscular architecture of the base comprises of a superficial (from lumen) longitudinal layer and a deep circular layer, which is continuous with the detrusor. The bladder neck assists in the maintenance of continence. In men, an anatomically definable circular smooth muscle is present; however, in women, no such muscle can be identified. Nevertheless, urethral pressure profilometry and videourodynamic studies have confirmed the presence of 'functional' bladder neck with circumferential compression in both the sexes (Figures 1A and B).

The muscles in relation to urethra are comprised of the following:
a. The urethral smooth muscle—in both the sexes, it is arranged in obvious layers, inner longitudinal (thicker) and outer circular (thinner).
b. Rhabdosphincter—this is the 'horse-shoe shaped' skeletal muscle layer within the wall of urethra and is separate from the 'pelvic floor periurethral

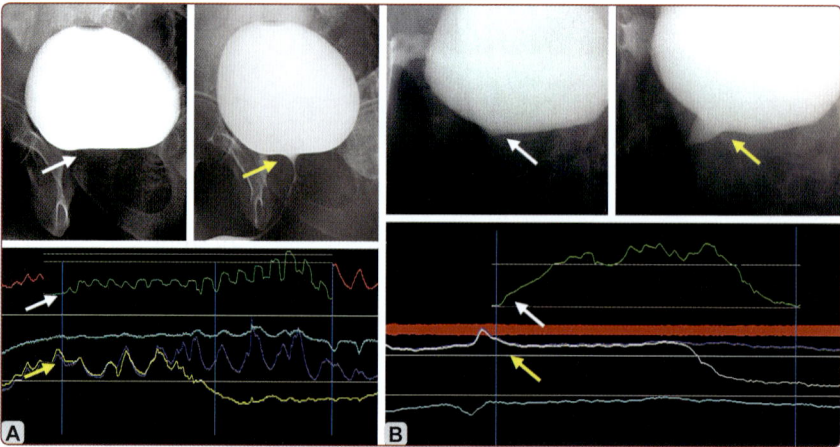

Figs 1A and B: Cystometry and urethral pressure profilometry depicting functional bladder neck (BN) in a male with symptomatic benign enlargement of prostate (A) and a female with pelvic floor dysfunction with non-relaxing external sphincter (B). White arrows point towards closed BN before micturition and yellow arrows to open BN during micturition. Green tracing depicts resting urethral pressure profile

muscles'. In males it is present from bladder base, through the prostate to all along the length of membranous urethra. In females, it extends from bladder neck downwards all along the length of urethra. The configuration of rhabdosphincter is depicted in Figures 2A to C.

c. Pelvic floor musculature—the disposition of levator ani complex muscles leaves a visceral hiatus anteriorly through which pelvic viscera, viz urethra and rectum in both the sexes and vagina in females. The part of the muscle-complex bordering these viscera is called 'pubovisceralis'.

Muscles of the pelvic floor are composed of both slow and fast twitch fibers, whereas the rhabdosphincter fibers are only the former type.

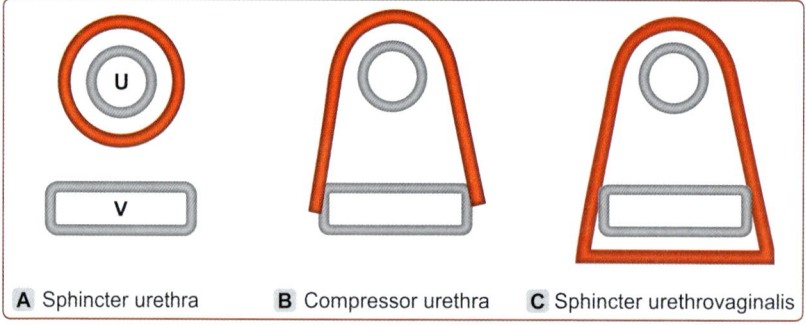

Figs 2A to C: Configuration of rhabdosphincter in females—(A) In the proximal urethra, it surrounds the urethra circumferentially (sphincter urethra); (B) In the mid-urethra, it is horse-shoe-shaped and fibers are inserted into the vaginal wall (compressor urethra); (C) In the distal urethra, it encircles the urethra and vagina (sphincter urethravaginalis)

FUNCTION OF THE LOWER URINARY TRACT

Primary function of the lower urinary tract is the storage of urine and maintenance of continence. To accomplish the storage function, bladder 'accommodates' a large volume of urine without increasing the luminal pressure. This requires rearrangement of collagen and elastin fibers, and reorientation of smooth muscles with distension. For the maintenance of continence, all the sphincters remain closed. Urethral pressure profilometry studies have shown maximum closure pressure in the region of external sphincter (rhabdosphincter and levator ani) [Figures 3A and B].

In addition to muscles, the mucosal folds and the cushioning effect of 'spongy' submucosa contribute variably to continence. In women, changes in hormonal milieu lead to atrophy of the 'sponge' increasing their risk for incontinence.

In addition to the above, other factors contributing to continence in women at times of increased abdominal pressure are as follows:

a. Proximal part of the urethra lies within the pelvic cavity and, therefore, during increased abdominal pressure, compression pressure from outside balances the downward pressure from the bladder (Figure 4).
b. *The Hammock:* Pelvic urethral support anteriorly by pubo-urethral ligaments, laterally by urethro-pelvic ligaments and posteriorly by pubocervical fascia (over the firm vaginal base) helps antero-posterior compression of the urethral walls during increased abdominal pressure (DeLancey's hammock hypothesis).
c. *The guarding reflex:* Intact nerve supply to the pelvic floor helps contraction of pelvic floor muscles in advance to direct transmission of abdominal pressure to the urethra.

Voiding function of LUT incorporates relaxation of all the sphincters followed by active detrusor contraction to empty the bladder. In women, opening of bladder neck and maintenance of optimum urethro-vesical angle is important for adequate bladder emptying. Fibro-muscular pelvic support is important in the latter function. In the presence of deficiency of pelvic-floor support, for

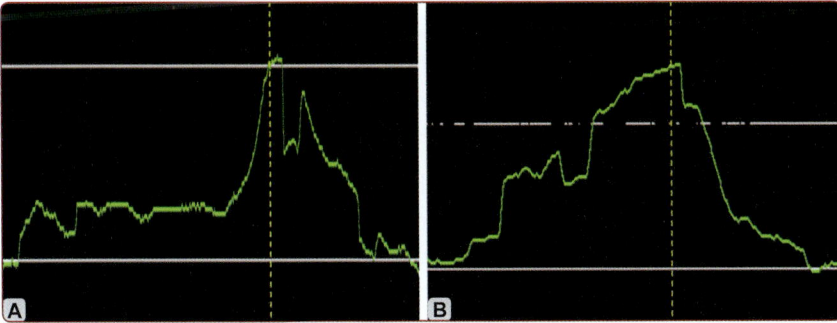

Figs 3A and B: Urethral pressure profilometry in the resting phase showing peak-pressure in the distal part, i.e. in the external sphincter zone (vertical broken line) in male (A) and female (B)

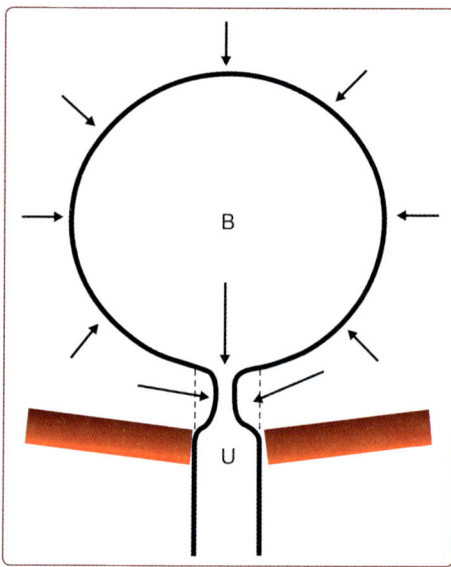

Fig. 4: The role of intrapelvic location of proximal part of female urethra in maintaining continence during rise in abdominal pressure. Downward vesical vector (B) is counterbalanced by transmission of Pabdominal to proximal urethra (inward arrows)

example, in the presence of advanced cystocele, bladder emptying may be severely compromised. The interested reader is advised to refer to excellent descriptions of PE Papa Petros.

NEURAL CONTROL OF THE LOWER URINARY TRACT

The LUT is innervated by sensory and motor, somatic (pudendal) as well as autonomic (pelvic and hypogastric) nervous system. The somatic supply is to the EUS and autonomic to bladder and urethral smooth muscles. The pelvic afferent myelinated and unmyelinated neurons respond to mechanical stretch of the bladder. During inflammatory conditions, recruitment of hitherto silent unmyelinated C-fibers in mucosa and muscles leads to 'hypersensitivity' and 'overactivity'.

Storage Phase

During the filling or storage phase, bladder distension reflexively generates the 'filling response' in the form of contraction of internal (sympathetic) and external (somatic) sphincter and detrusor inactivity (parasympathetic silence). With continued filling, in the presence of socially appropriate circumstances, heightened afferent discharge from bladder stimulates detrusor contraction (parasympathetic) coupled with sympathetic and somatic inactivity. Pontine micturition center coordinates this switch-over; lesions affecting pontine control (e.g. cervico-dorsal spinal injuries) lead to 'detrusor-sphincter dyssynergia' in which detrusor and sphincters contract at the same time leading to voiding dysfunction and pose a threat to the upper tracts.

Reflexes in the Storage Phase

a. *Bladder to urethra reflex*—distension of bladder stimulates central pathways such that sympathetic efferents as well as pudendal efferents are stimulated, resulting in internal and external sphincteric contraction, respectively. It is seen on electromyography as progressively increasing amplitude with filling (Figure 5).
b. *Urethra to bladder reflex*—EUS contraction or contraction of anal sphincter, stimulation from vagina, rectum and perineum inhibit the voiding function through the centrally mediated pathways.

Voiding Phase

There is 'switch' of activities which initiate micturition. At the micturition threshold, continued afferent activity from the bladder reverses the activity of the efferent pathway.
- Silence of somatic motor system: relaxation of external sphincter
- Silence of sympathetic system: relaxation of bladder neck sphincter
- Stimulation of parasympathetic system: detrusor contraction and relaxation of bladder neck sphincter (through the release of NO).

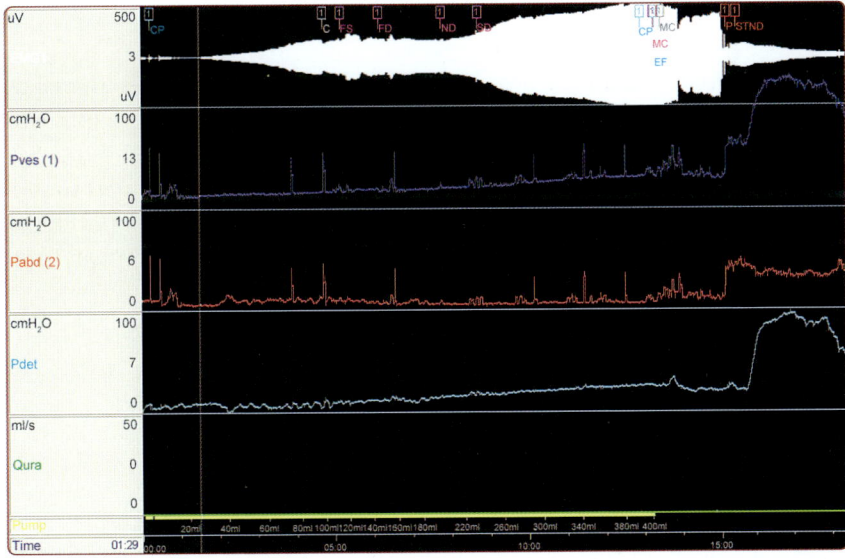

Fig. 5: EMG tracing during the filling phase showing progressively increasing EMG activity with progressive filling of bladder (guarding reflex). Sudden relative silence of EMG activity represents sphincteric relaxation with the initiation of the micturitional phase

Reflexes in the Voiding Phase

Urethra to bladder reflex: Urine in the urethra stimulates detrusor contraction; this cascade promotes complete bladder emptying.

The coordination of parasympathetic activity and sympathetic/somatic silence is performed at Pontine Micturition Center (eponymed as Barrington's nucleus). The afferent bladder activity for the 'switch' is relayed to the PMC through midbrain's PAG region.

Lesions of PMC or disconnection below the PMC lead to detrusor-sphincter dyssynergia.

Voluntary control on micturition depends on the connections of frontal cortex, hypothalamus and brainstem.

Lesions of these regions of cortex and hypothalamus lead to the loss of voluntary control on micturition as well as lead to detrusor overactivity.

SUGGESTED READING

1. Papa Petros PE. The Female Pelvic Floor: Function, Dysfunction and Management According to the Integral Theory. Second Edition. Heidelberg: Springer Medizin Verlag; 2007.

CHAPTER 2

Clinical Assessment of a Patient with Lower Urinary Tract Symptoms

Voiding dysfunction is a conglomerate of various lower urinary tract symptoms; it can be of varied etiology. A careful comprehensive history and detailed examination is the key to rational diagnosis and successful treatment. However, it must be emphasized that inasmuch as clinically useful, history can be misleading and examination may be unremarkable. A classic example is a patient of chronic retention and obstructive nephropathy presenting with decreased appetite, nocturnal incontinence and otherwise minimal LUTS; a palpable bladder and enlarged prostate often will clinch the diagnosis.

It is useful to follow a proforma-based clinical assessment to avoid missing significant information on history and examination. The following specific points should not be excluded in history and examination and, therefore, be included in the proforma.

HISTORY

Lower Urinary Tract Symptoms (LUTS)

- *Storage symptoms*—frequency, urgency, nocturia
- *Voiding symptoms*—hesitancy, intermittency, poor stream, sensation of incomplete evacuation, straining at micturition, post-void dribbling, terminal dribbling
- *Incontinence*—with urgency, with abdominal straining, while walking, continuous, enuresis, uncharacterizable
- *Characterization of urgency*—for pain/burning or for fear of leakage. *This is very useful in understanding the underlying pathology, whether inflammation or overactivity, respectively.*
- *Hematuria*—total, terminal, initial, urethral hemorrhage, painless or painful
- Dysuria, urethral discharge.

Pain

- *Location*—suprapubic, low-back, perineum, rectum, introitus, vagina, pelvis
- Pain/burning during ejaculation (male) or vaginal intercourse (female)
- Back pain, limb pain/weakness

Other Processes which may Affect LUT Function

- *Injury/surgery*—Urinary tract (e.g. traumatic catheterization, pelvic fracture, straddle injury), peripheral nerves (e.g. radical hysterectomy, abdomino-perineal resection), spinal cord, brain
- *Disease*—e.g. diabetes mellitus (polyuria or neuropathy), parkinsonism, cebrebrovascular accident, prolapsed intervertebral disc, vertebral deformity
- *Medication*—e.g. diuretics, calcium channel blockers, alpha blockers, anticholinergics, anti-histaminics, selective serotonin or serotonin-norepinephrine reuptake inhibitors, dopaminergics, thyroxine.

Urinary Tract Infection

Recurrent/infrequent; with fever/without fever.

Defecation

Constipation (decreased sensation or difficulty in evacuation), fecal/gas urgency, incontinence.

Other Symptoms

- High-risk sexual contact, e.g. multiple partners, commercial sex-worker, non-vaginal intercourse (oral, anal, etc.)
- Menstrual history, history of child-birth, discharge
- Symptoms other than referred to pelvis/LUT, e.g. abdominal pain, dyspeptic symptoms, past/present history of tuberculosis.

EXAMINATION

Abdominal—Mass, surgical scar, hepato-splenomegaly, bladder, hernia

Male-specific

- *Genital*—penis, meatus, testes, epididymis
- *Digital rectal*—perineum, prostate—size/consistency, mass in rectum or cul-de-sac, bimanual (if appropriate)
- *Focused neurological*—perianal sensations, anal tone (normal, decreased or increased), bulbocavernosus reflex (pinching glans, pull on catheter), voluntary anal contraction and relaxation
- *Lower limb reflexes*—knee, ankle, plantar.

Female-specific

Focused neurological and digital rectal similar to male (except for prostate).

Pelvic Examination

- Clitoris—phimosis
- Meatus—aperture, caruncle, mucosal prolapse
- Vagina—estrogenic condition, discharge, fistula, mass
- Incontinence—urethral, vaginal.

Pelvic Support Defect (Figure 1)

Level I: Uterine/vault prolapse, enterocele.

Level II: Anterior—cystocele; paravaginal or central
Posterior—rectocele; enterocele.

Level III: Anterior—urethral hypermobility
Posterior—descent of perineal body.

Bladder Diary

Bladder diary or *urolog* is a superior method of recording the history of drinking habit and LUTS than the recall-based history. The longer it is kept, the more useful it is; nevertheless, it is reasonable to keep a 48-hour log (Figure 3). A comprehensive diary would contain information on all of the following:
a. Fluid intake—timing, quality and quantity
b. Urine output—timing and quantity

A		P
Enterocele Y/N Stage_____	Uterine/Vault Y/N Stage_____ Level-I	Enterocele Y/N Stage_____
Cystocele Y/N Stage_____ Paravaginal y/n Central y/n	Level-II	Rectocele Y/N Stage_____
Urethral Hypermobility Y/N Degree_____	Level-III	Perineal descent Y/N Stage_____

Fig. 1: Pelvic support defect schemata

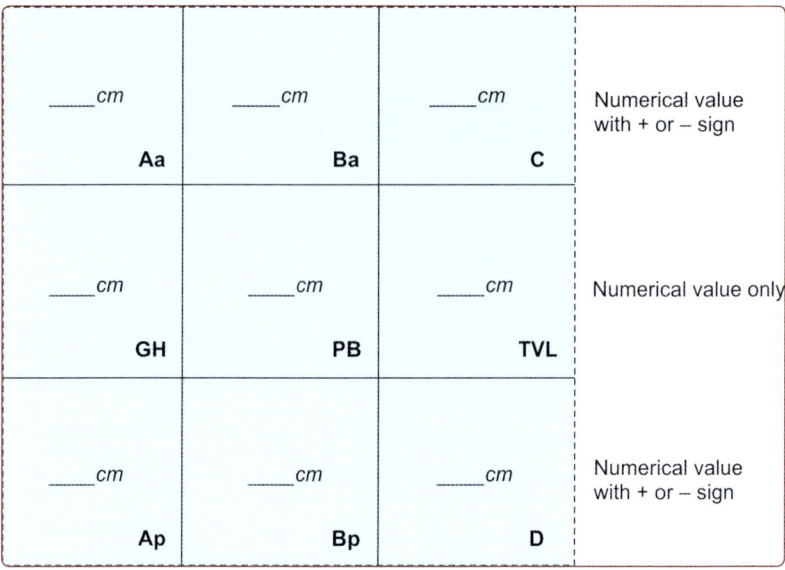

Fig. 2: Standardized pelvic-floor prolapsed Quantification system

c. Timing, qualification and grading of other symptoms, e.g. urgency, pain and incontinence.

Naturally, a comprehensive urolog would be helpful in answering the following queries:

a. Whether the patient has polyuria (defined as daily output of >40 mL/kg); whether there is nocturnal polyuria.
b. Whether the patient has urgency for pain, leak or both.
c. Whether there is incontinence; if yes, what type and how much.
d. What type of diurnal frequency does the patient have—fixed volume (suggestive of inflammatory/fibrotic process; hypersensate bladder) or variable volume (suggestive of overactivity).
e. Whether there is nocturia–often patients with overactive bladder do not have nocturia; however, patients with hypersensate bladder will be bothered with nocturia.
f. Functional bladder capacity (FBC): helps to determine appropriate fill rate during multichannel urodynamics, if required (e.g. an appropriate fill rate would be 5–10% of FBC per minute).

Apart from quantification of symptoms, it helps the clinician to understand the underlying pathology and also design an individualized behavioral modification, scheduled-voiding plan. A follow-up log helps both the physician and the patient to understand the response to therapy. In our experience, we have had patients pinpoint diagnosed just on the basis of urology. An extreme example is given as follows:

Chapter 2 Clinical Assessment of a Patient with Lower Urinary Tract Symptoms

BLADDEER DIARY

Department of urology, Postgraduate Institute of Medical Education and Research, Chandigarh, India

Date	Day 1			Day 2		
	Drinks		Urine	Drinks		Urine
	What?	How much? (ml)	How much? (ml)	What?	How much? (ml)	How much? (ml)
Sample						
6-7 AM						
7-8 AM						
8-9 AM						
9-10 AM						
10-11 AM						
11-12 PM						
12-1 PM						
1-2 PM						
2-3 PM						
3-4 PM						
4-5 PM						
5-6 PM						
6-7 PM						
7-8 PM						
8-9 PM						
9-10 PM						
10-11 PM						
11-12 MN						
12-1 AM						
1-2 AM						
2-3 AM						
3-4 AM						
4-5 AM						
5-6 AM						

- Choose a 3 days' period to keep this record when you can conveniently measure your voids.
- If you are unable to keep the diary for a 24-hour period, try to keep it for as many hours as possible.
- Include all voids, even if they occur in the middle of the night.
- Underline each void accompanied by abnormal urgency (a sudden compelling desire to void which is diffcult to postpone).
- If you leak urine, please wear pad all the time during the days of bladder diary. Record the number of soaked pads you had to change during each day. Note your activity at the time of any leakage.
- Enter the following marks in the box when you have an accidental leakage of urine (even the slightest amount).
- "U" because you could not make it to toilet, "S" during cough, sneeze, laugh, physical exertion, straining or activity. "W" without knowing.
- Enter "P" in the box when you feel pain which you think is related to your bladder (pain in lower belly, urinary passage, and pain on filling of bladder).
- Mark the box you went to bed at night and you woke up in the morning finally.

Fig. 3: Bladder diary in use at PGIMER, Chandigarh

A 43-year-old man with no other comorbidity presented with urinary frequency day and night. He did not have any significant urgency or voiding symptoms. His initial workup revealed creatinine 0.74 mg/dL, hemoglobin—15.3 g/dL and a normal urine examination. Ultrasound revealed bilateral moderate hydroureteronephrosis with large capacity thick-walled bladder and 150 mL post-void urine. Uroflowmetry revealed Qmax 39 mL/sec, voided volume—990 mL, PVR—205 mL and normal voiding pattern. To our surprise, his urolog showed the following findings:

❖ Daily fluid intake 24,400 mL
❖ Daily urine output 23,900 mL

- Functional bladder capacity—1100 mL
- Day-time frequency—17 (volume 800–1000 mL)
- Night-time frequency—7 (volume 1000–1100 mL)
- Urgency—negative; pain—negative

He was a case of compulsive drinking and he was successfully managed with behavioral modification. Daily intake at last follow-up was 4 liters and hydroureteronephrosis had disappeared.

Although appealing, a comprehensive log is difficult to comply with. Therefore, often clinicians advise their patients to keep a frequency-volume chart or even only frequency chart. If the patient cannot keep a full 48-hour chart, he/she is encouraged to keep it as much as possible.

CHAPTER 3

Uroflowmetry

Uroflowmetry is a simple and useful measure of urine flow characteristics of an individual. Its importance lies in its non-invasiveness, and ease of performance and interpretation. The equipment is relatively simple and inexpensive. The initial thought of objective assessment of strength of urinary stream dates back to early 20th century, when Havelock Ellis (1902) attempted to describe urinary flow in terms of cast distance of the urinary stream. The first description of formal uroflowmeter with graphical representation is attributed to Willard M Drake, Jr (1946) followed by von Garrelts (1956) who emphasized that flow rates are dependent on voided volume.

Uroflowmetry is the measure of urine flow rate over time (Figure 1) and represents the final outcome of bladder function and status of bladder-outlet.

Flow measurements depend on various factors, e.g. voided volume, age, sex, voiding position, body mass index (in women), natural habits, and overall comfort during the measurement and psychological inhibition.

Hence, it is relevant and rather important to ask at the end of the void whether the uroflow was 'representative' of their natural act of voiding. Estimation of post-void residual urine by ultrasound is an important part of the uroflowmetry. It will be discussed in detail in the later section.

> **Tips**
> - It is not uncommon to come across patients who find it difficult to 'perform' uroflow in unfamiliar surroundings, typically a busy, noisy out-patient clinic. Therefore, for correct interpretation of uroflow, it is of utmost importance to explain the procedure to the patient, have clean, quiet and conducive environment for the void and provision for all three common voiding positions (i.e. standing, sitting and squatting), at least the former two.
> - Another important requirement often missed is adequately filled bladder. The patient should not be pushed to perform uroflow in haste, i.e. with underfilled bladder (which is likely to give insufficient information), nor should he/she be made to drink excessively or to wait too long for a 'really good' uroflow; in the latter scenario, patients often develop pain or uncomfortable urge to void which is not representative of their natural act.

- The patient should be asked to perform voiding in his/her preferred voiding position. Position related changes have been studied extensively but without consensus; however, many authors have emphasized the importance of 'natural voiding position' in this regard. For example, if we ask a woman who has always voided/passed stools in squatting position, to perform uroflowmetry in sitting position, the results are likely to be non-representative.
- The patient should be adequately counseled that he/she is not supposed to 'perform' uroflowmetry. Rather, they should take it as a routine representative voiding act. Few important considerations in this regard, which need to be excluded from a void, are:
  - Patients may be straining unusually to give us their 'best' performance
  - Male patients with voiding symptoms often develop habit of 'squeeze and release' of penis during voiding. In this way, urine is collected in anterior urethra and suddenly released, resulting in a 'reassuringly' high flow.
  - Cruising: Ideally, urine should fall on one area of the funnel without cruising around. Artifactually high peaks may be observed if urine flows directly into the central hole of the funnel or the patients move the stream around.

TYPES OF UROFLOWMETERS

1. *Gravimetric (weight transducer):* It operates by measuring the weight of collected fluid or by measuring the hydrostatic pressure at the base of collecting cylinder.
2. *Rotating disk method:* Urine flow is directed onto a rotating disk, increasing the inertia of the disk. The power needed to keep the disk rotating at a constant speed is measured and is proportional to the flow rate of the fluid.
3. *Electronic dipstick method:* It uses a capacitance dipstick mounted on the collecting chamber that changes its capacitance as urine accumulates in the cylinder. The output signal is proportional to the accumulated volume of urine.
4. *Magnetic (integral trap magnetic uroflowmeter):* Urine flowing through a magnetic field generates voltage proportional to flow rate.

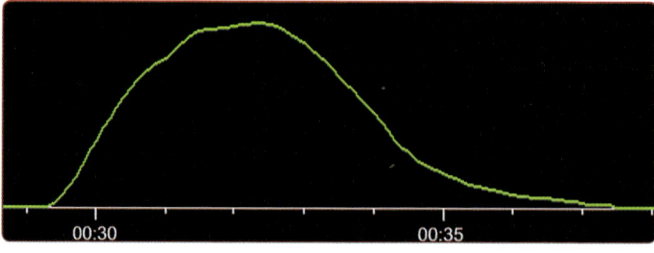

Fig. 1: Normal uroflow pattern—bell-shaped curve

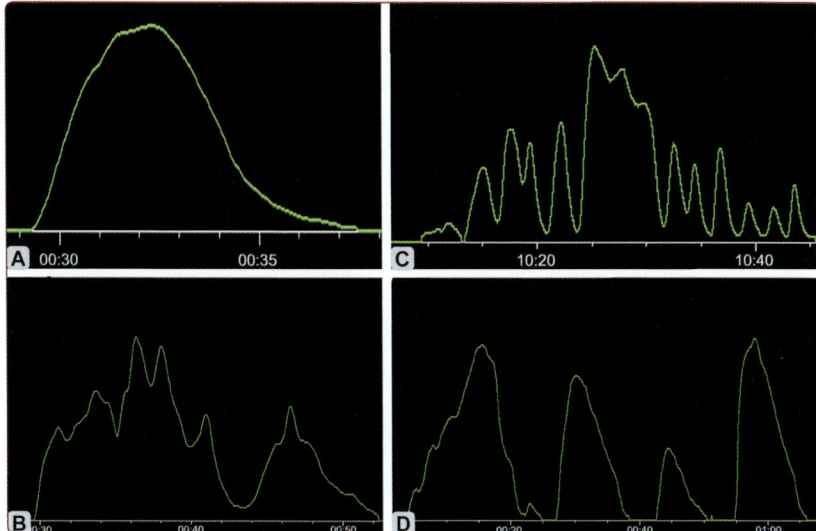

Figs 2A to D: Some uroflow patterns: (A) Normal; (B) Straining (irregular saw toothing); (C) Cruising (take a note of sharp peaks); (D) Squeezing (regular peaks)

One may acquire any of the types of uroflowmeter mentioned herewith. However, it is important to insure accuracy, safety and performance of the equipment as well as availability of after-sales service by the company. The desired clinical accuracy may differ from the technical accuracy of a flow meter.

STANDARDIZATION REQUIREMENTS OF THE EQUIPMENT

The ICS technical report recommended the following standards: a range of 0–50 mL/s for Qmax, and 0–1,000 mL for voided volume, maximum time constant of 0.75 s; an accuracy of + 5% relative to full scale, although a calibration curve representing the percentage error over the entire range of measurement should be made available. Full details of the standardization can be downloaded from the *ICS website—http://icsoffice.org/Documents/Documents.aspx?DocumentID=1*.

Setup

Typically, simple non-invasive uroflowmetry does not require an elaborate setup and it can actually be setup in a toilet. It is rather desirable to have the uroflowmetry room resemble a clean toilet (Figure 3).

It should be clean, quiet, cool, adequately lit and conveniently located and lockable from inside. It should preferably have a wash-basin. Various types of chairs are available, ranging from simple western commode-like chair (Figure 3) to the most advanced electromechanical chairs (Figure 4). The latter are typically a part of invasive multichannel UDS unit rather than simple uroflowmetry. Nevertheless, the latter are helpful in making squatting position.

The essential parts of a uroflowmeter are as follows (Figure 5):
- Base-plate, the basic measurement transducer
- Beaker, the receptacle for urine
- Funnel
- Stand
- Connections
- Processor
- Printout
- Wired/wireless.

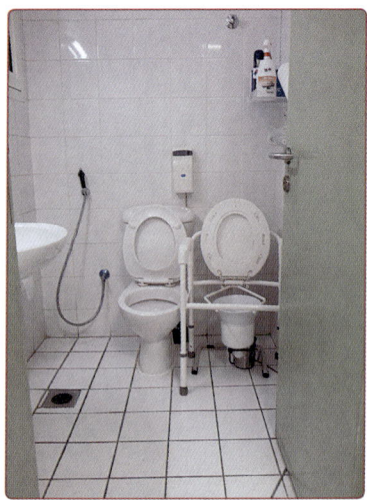

Fig. 3: Uroflowmetry setup at New Medical Center Specialty Hospital, Abu Dhabi, UAE

HOW TO READ AND INTERPRET UROFLOW DATA

Measurements

The following measurements are recommended by the ICS during uroflowmetry (Figure 6):

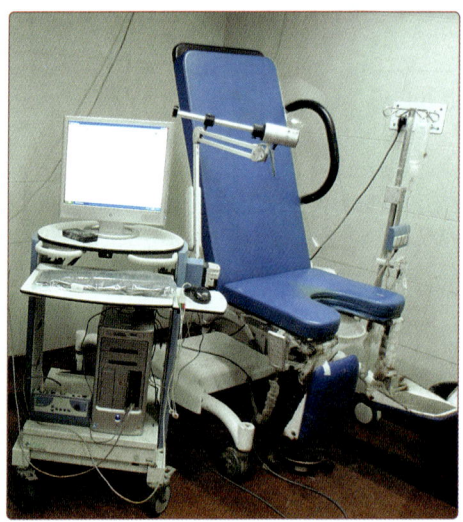

Fig. 4: Urodynamic setup of PGIMER, Chandigarh, India with electromechanical fluoroscopy-compatible urodynamic chair (Sonesta)

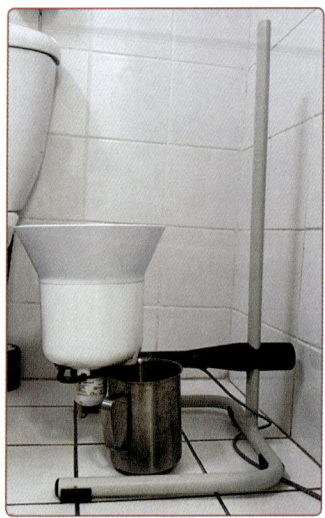

Fig. 5: Parts of a uroflowmeter

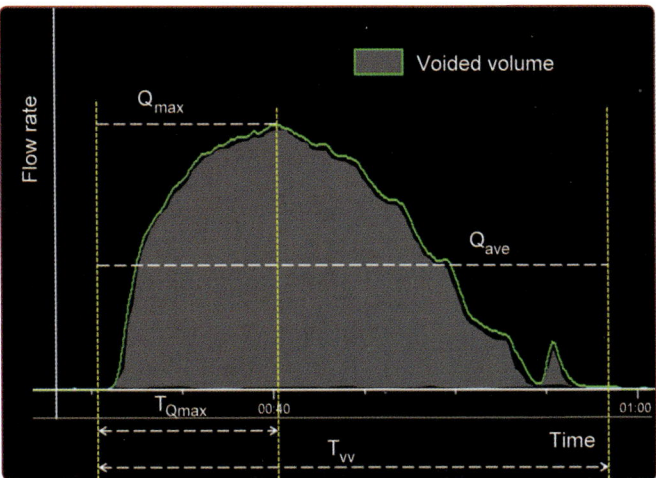

Fig. 6: Analysis of uroflowmetry graph

- *Flow rate (Q; mL/sec):* It is the amount of fluid (urine) expelled out of urethra per unit time. The following two flow-rates are specifically mentioned:
  - *Maximum flow rate (Qmax):* It is the maximum measured value of Q. It is generally reached by initial 1/3rd of volume. However, variations are quite common.
  - *Average flow rate (Qave):* It is the average representation of the whole flow, i.e. voided volume/flow time. It's value is generally half of Qmax. However, in intermittent flow states, this relation differs and Qave < ½ Qmax. In calculating Qave in intermittent flow, time without flow is disregarded.
- *Voided volume (VV; mL):* It is the total volume of urine/fluid collected into the uroflow-beaker. Please note that any urine not collecting in the beaker is not measured by the flowmeter and this may significantly affect the calculation of flow rates.
- *Flow time (Tvv; sec):* Time over which measureable flow occurs. In intermittent flow, time without flow is subtracted from the total voiding time to give flow-time. In continuous flow, voiding time equals flow time.
- *Time to Qmax (TQmax; sec):* Time taken from start of flow to Qmax. It is generally about 1/3rd of flow time, but may vary. In our separate studies on healthy men and women, mean and standard deviation of these values were 30.9±12.3% and 36.7±15.5% respectively.

Flow Patterns (Figures 7A to E)

Careful study of flow pattern can assist the numerical information in the interpretation of uroflowmetry. The following patterns are described:

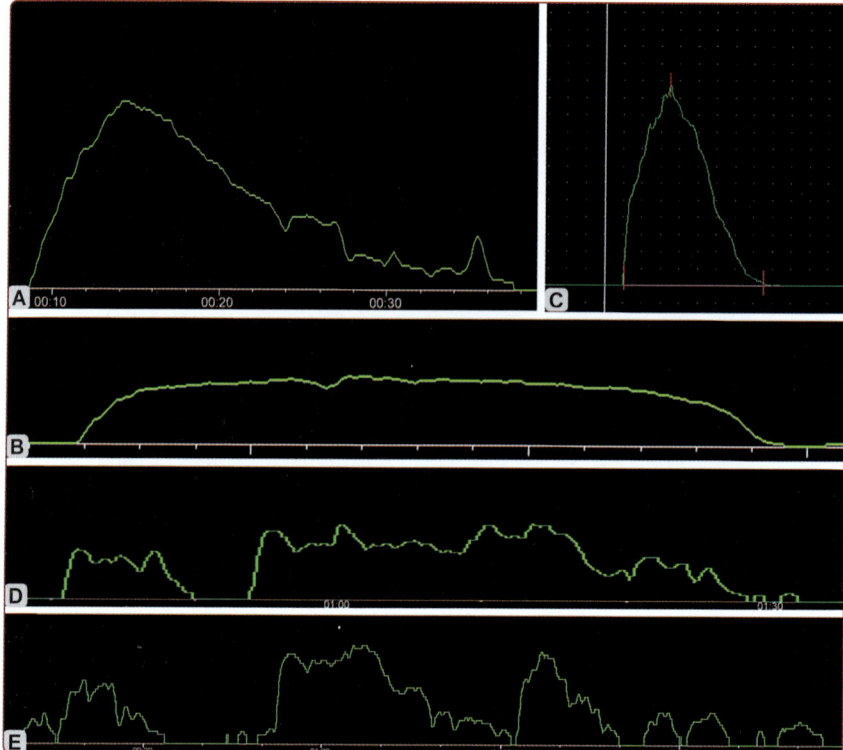

Figs 7A to E: Some recognized abnormal uroflow-patterns. (A) Compressive obstruction; (B) Constrictive obstruction; (C) Overactive bladder; (D) Detrusor underactivity; (E) Intermittent voiding pattern

a. *Normal:* It is a bell-shaped curve (meso-kurtotic type) with Qmax reached in initial 1/3rd of the void (usually 3–10 seconds); however, significant variations may be observed depending on various factors.
b. Bladder outlet obstruction:
   ➢ *Compressive*, e.g. benign prostatic hyperplasia or bladder neck obstruction. Pattern of initial part of void till Qmax may seem normal, but there is terminal prolongation. Qave is generally more than half of Qmax.
   ➢ *Constrictive*, e.g. urethral stricture. A low Qmax is rapidly reached and flow rate remains relatively constant at that, giving a box-like or plateau-shaped appearance. There is no significant difference between Qmax and Qave.
c. *Detrusor Overactivity:* Peaked type of flow pattern (leptokurtotic) abnormally high Qmax are reached in unusually short time (<3 seconds). This happens due to high contraction velocities of the detrusor.

d. *Detrusor Underactivity:* This low pressure, low flow pattern is very variable with Qmax generally reached by half-way or even in the second half of the void. There can be a significant overlap with obstructed patterns.
e. *Intermittent:* The flow is not continuous; the uroflow shows an interrupted pattern. Generally, straining in the presence of poor or absent detrusor contraction gives saw-toothed appearance with relatively fixed height of each flow (signifying similar amplitude of abdominal straining).

Intermittent flow due to high grade prostatic obstruction generally is not associated with straining and has more crescendo-decrescendo pattern.

Postvoid Residual Urine (PVRU)

It is important to measure PVRU immediately after uroflowmetry. This indicates the status of detrusor function with respect to the outlet resistance, whether bladder outlet obstruction (BOO) or detrusor underactivity (DUA). It can be measured effectively by abdominal ultrasonography. Volume estimations vary depending upon the shape of the bladder, which is even more important in PVRU, where the shape is more of a squashed football. However, for practical purposes, the formula D1 X D2 X D3 X 0.7 gives a reasonable estimate of PVRU; whereas, D1 and D2 are mutually perpendicular diameters in sagittal plane and D3 transverse diameter in coronal plane. Automated bladder-scanners designed for the measurement of PVRU come in handy for this purpose (Figure 8). Finally, one must understand that ultrasound gives only an estimate based on formulae which may vary widely from the actual measurement.

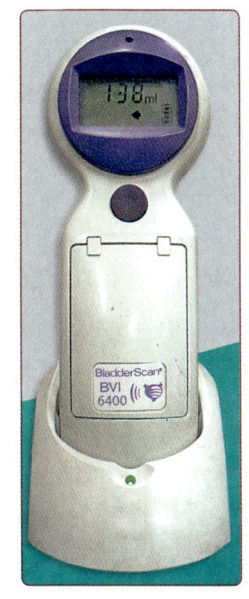

Fig. 8: Hand-held bladder scan

Obviously, the most accurate measurement of PVRU is by urethral catheterization. It carries a risk of introducing infection, particularly in men. Therefore, it is permissible only in circumstances when the patient already does periodic self-catheterization (e.g. orthotopic neobladder, detrusor underactivity) or the free-uroflowmetry is to be immediately followed by an invasive multichannel UDS.

The above description pertains to the performance of uroflowmetry and acquisition of numerical and graphical information. The following discussion concentrates on how to interpret this information:

We recollect from the introduction that the most important determinant of uroflow rates in a given individual is voided volume. Therefore, before declaring any uroflow abnormal, information of voided volume is essential. For example, a Qmax of 15 mL/sec may be considered subnormal at a VV of 400 mL; however, it would be within the normal range at 150 mL. There are a couple of ways to objectively interpret Qmax and Qave in relation to VV.

Flow-volume Nomograms

These are the curves plotted between Q (y-axis) and VV (x-axis) and represent distribution of normal Q-VV relations. Various nomograms are available for both the sexes and different age groups. Of these, Siroky and Liverpool nomograms for adult men and Liverpool nomograms for adult women have been in common use worldwide (Figures 9A to D).

We have observed that normal Q-VV relations in our population (both men and women) are below par compared to these nomograms. We developed and validated nomograms based on local north Indian population which are eponymed as PGIMER nomograms (Figures 10A to D).

We have found that the lower 68% confidence limit line in each of these nomograms gives a reasonable cut-off for abnormal flow, requiring further investigations. Moreover, any value above median line represents essentially normal flow.

Volume Corrected Q

Another concept useful to correctly interpret uroflow is volume corrected flow rate (cQ) or flow-volume index (VQI). It is defined differently for men and women as follows:

- $cQ^* = Q/\sqrt{BV}$ (for men in standing and squatting position and women in sitting position)

  * Qmax or Qave. BV (bladder volume) = VV + PVR
- cQ is conceptually similar to body mass index (BMI); BMI = weight (Kg)/[height (m)]^2. We know that BMI is a well accepted derivation of weight and height and used instead of either for defining and categorizing obesity. Similarly, cQ can be utilized in defining voiding dysfunction. The reference values of flow rates and corrected flow rates in Indian population are as follows:

	Men	Women
Qmax	24.1 ± 7.9	23.5 ± 9.3
Qave	13.9 ± 4.8	13.3 ± 6.0
cQmax	1.41 ± 0.44	1.44 ± 0.42
cQave	0.80 ± 0.28	0.81 ± 0.27

Indications can be broadly classified into:
- *Screening:* for voiding dysfunction in patients presenting with voiding type LUTS irrespective of etiology (e.g. benign prostatic hyperplasia, bladder neck dysfunction, pelvic floor spasticity, neurogenic bladder)

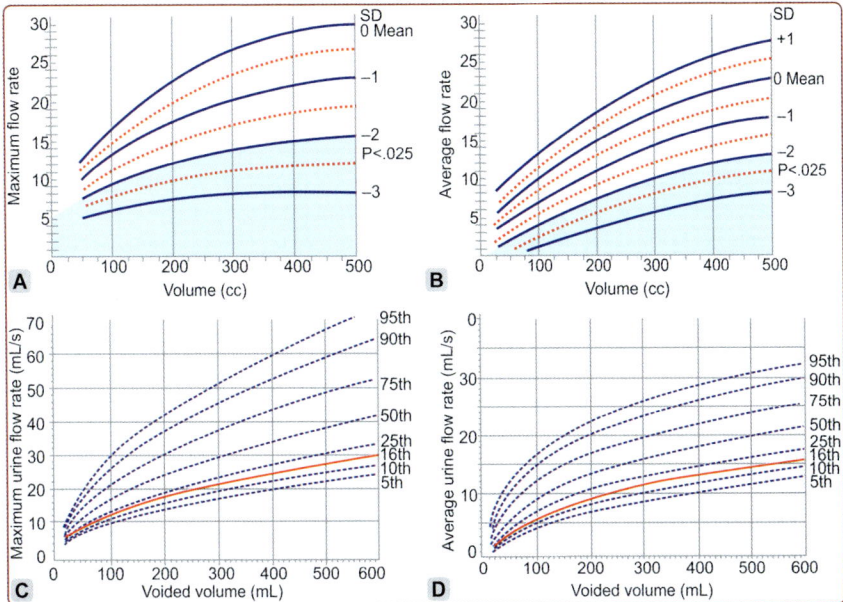

Figs 9A to D: Flow volume nomograms developed on Caucasian population. Siroky nomograms for men—Qmax-VV (A), Qave-VV (B); Liverpool nomograms for women—Qmax-VV (C), Qave-VV (D)

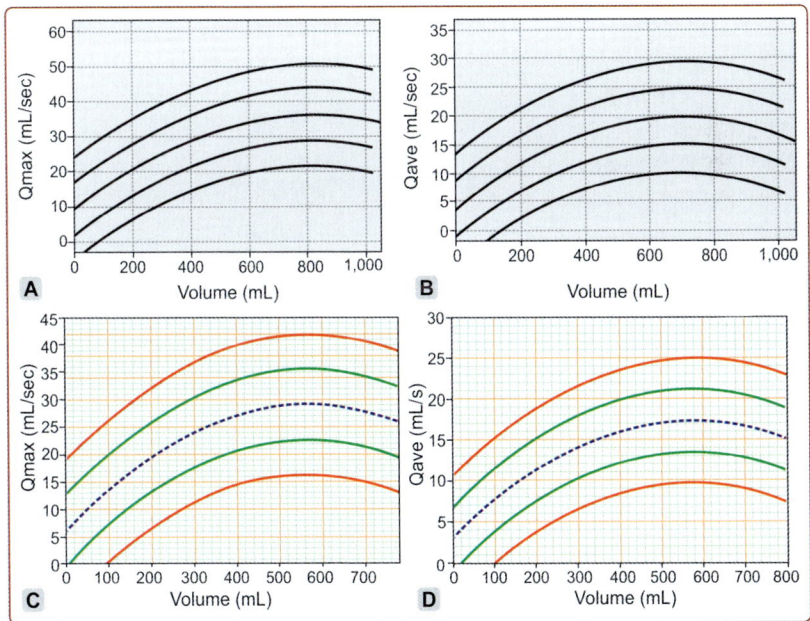

Figs 10A to D: PGIMER flow-volume nomograms developed on Indian population for women (A and B) and men (C and D)

❖ *Evaluation of clinical response:* To the medical/surgical management of above conditions.

SUGGESTED READING

1. Agarwal MM, Shivkumar SP, Roy K, et al. Rationalization of interpretation of Uroflowmetry for a non-Caucasian (Indian) population: development and validation of volume-normalized flow rate index and flow-volume nomograms. Neurourol Urodynam. 2013. [Epub ahead of print]
2. Barapatre Y, Agarwal MM, Singh SK, Sharma SK, Mavuduru RM, Mete UK, et al. Uroflowmetry in healthy women: development and validation of flow—volume and corrected flow—age nomograms. Neurourol Urodynam. 2009;28(8):1003–9.
3. Haylen BT, Ashby D, Sutherst JR, Frazer MI, West CR. Maximum and average urine flow rates in normal male and female populations—The Liverpool nomograms. Br J Urol. 1989;64:30–8.
4. Siroky MB, Olessen CA, Krane RJ. The flow rate nomogram in development. J Urol. 1979;122:665–8.

CHAPTER
4
Cystometry and Pressure-flow Study

HARDWARE

Base Unit

Urodynamics is a computer-based investigation which comprises of hardware for acquisition of data and software to analyze and compute it. Acquisition of data is sent to computer program via transducers, which essentially converts physical energy into electrical signals from various peripheral portals. The following portals are commonly used:

1. Signals from bladder: pressure in the bladder (Pves).
2. Signals from abdomen: pressure in the abdomen measured in one of the following—rectum/vagina/abdominal bowel diversion (Pabd).
3. Signals from pelvic floor muscles (EMG).
4. Signals from uroflowmeter
   - Flow (Qura)
   - Volume (Vvoid).
5. Signals from pump: infused volume (Vinf).
6. Signals from puller: length of urethral profile.

Catheters

These are used to acquire pressure signals from bladder (Pves) and abdomen (Pabd). Three types of catheters are clinically used:

a. *Fluid-infused catheter:* The principle of pressure measurement with a continuously infused open-ended catheter in a closed organ is that mechanical force from the organ is transferred to a fluid pressure in the catheter through a liquid column to an external transducer. These are the most commonly used worldwide. These catheters can be single lumen (rectal pressure), double lumen (bladder pressure) or triple lumen (bladder and urethral pressure); in the latter two, one lumen is designated for fluid infusion (Figures 1A to C).

b. *Air-charged balloon catheter:* This catheter consists of a channel for fluid instillation and one or two miniature circumferential balloons which are

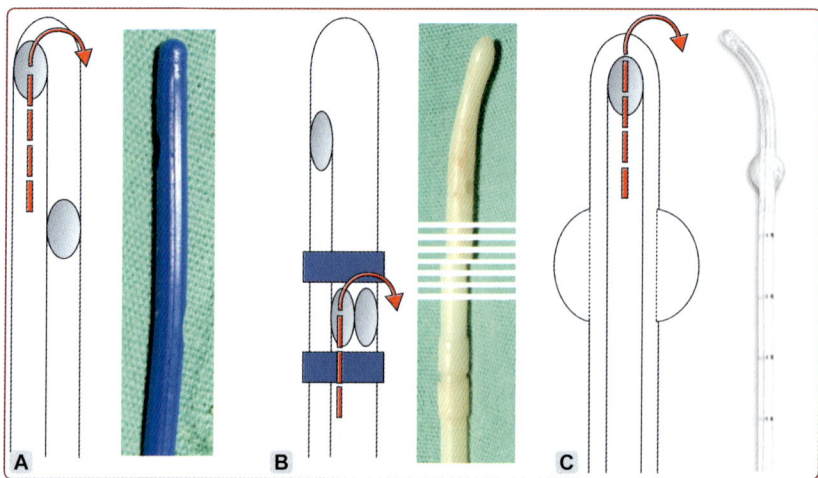

Figs 1A to C: Internal anatomy of tips of UDS catheters—(A) Two-lumen cystometry catheter: perfusion channel orifice at the tip (curved arrow), Pves channel orifice 1 cm proximal to it; (B) Three-lumen UPP catheter: Pves channel orifice at the tip, perfusion channel orifice (curved arrow) adjacent to Pura channel orifice 5 cm proximal to Pves. Circular border on either side of the proximal orifices insures proper pressure measurement by Pura; (C) Double-lumen air-charged cystometry catheter: perfusion channel orifice at the tip (curved arrow), Pves channel balloon 1 cm proximal to it. To note, three-lumen UPP catheter has perfusion channel orifice at the tip and Pves and Pura channel-balloons 1 and 6 cm proximal to it, respectively

connected to an external transducer especially designed for these catheters. The balloons are 'air-charged' through a mechanism in the transducer and the pressure of the balloon's location is transmitted to the transducer. These offer the following advantages over the above type catheters:
   i. Studies have shown that the measurements from this catheter system is remarkably consistent compared to fluid-infused or micro-tip transducer type catheter systems.[1,2]
   ii. This system is capable of circumferential measurement of pressure and superior response time leading to smoother tracings.[2]
   iii. These catheter transducers can be integrated into existing urodynamic systems.

   Currently, the largest manufacturer and supplier of these catheters is T-DOC® Company, LLC, Wilmington, DE *(<http://www.tdocllc.com/index2.php>)*.

c. *Catheter-mounted microtransducers:* These are reusable sterilizable catheters with miniature transducers mounted on the tip of catheter. These are connected to a computer via cables. Unlike fixed external transducers, which can be zeroed to a particular level (i.e. pubic symphysis), the catheter-mounted transducer cannot be zeroed to a specific level, since the tip is mobile in the bladder.

Electrodes

In many circumstances, it is useful and important to know functional status of electrical activity of pelvic floor, or sometimes, more specifically external urethral sphincter. For example, increased sphincteric activity during micturitional phase in detrusor sphincter dysynnergia, non-relaxation of external sphincter in dysfunctional elimination syndrome and bizarre repetitive discharges in sphincteric motor units in Fowler's syndrome. Simple kinesiologic electromyography (EMG), i.e. study of amplitude and frequency is all that is required in most circumstances and can be performed using non-invasive surface electrodes, luminal electrodes (vaginal) or by more invasive concentric needle electrodes (Figures 2A to C).

Both external anal and urethral sphincters relax during micturition. Therefore, in most circumstances, surface electrodes placed by either side of anus are able to give clinically meaningful results (Figures 3A to F).

Care should be taken to make the perianal area clean and dry, and place the electrodes securely close to anus, since this area has minimal fat even in most obese patients.

Introduction

- Uroflow cannot differentiate obstruction/weak detrusor.
- Importance of knowing in what is happening 'inside'.
- History of PFS.

Setup/Equipment

Bedside 'single channel' simple cystometry has been a common practice in which fluid is filled through a urethral catheter and the patient is asked to

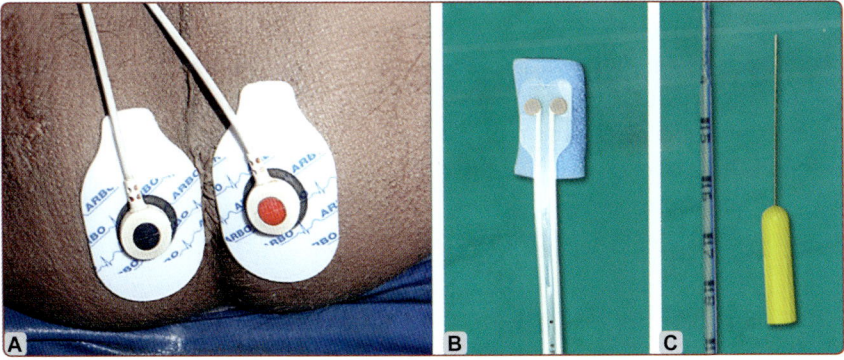

Figs 2A to C: Electromyography electrodes. (A) Surface perineal electrodes—to be placed as close to anus as possible; (B) Vaginal sponge electrode; (C) Concentric needle electrode for direct sphincteric EMG measurement

26 Manual of Urodynamics

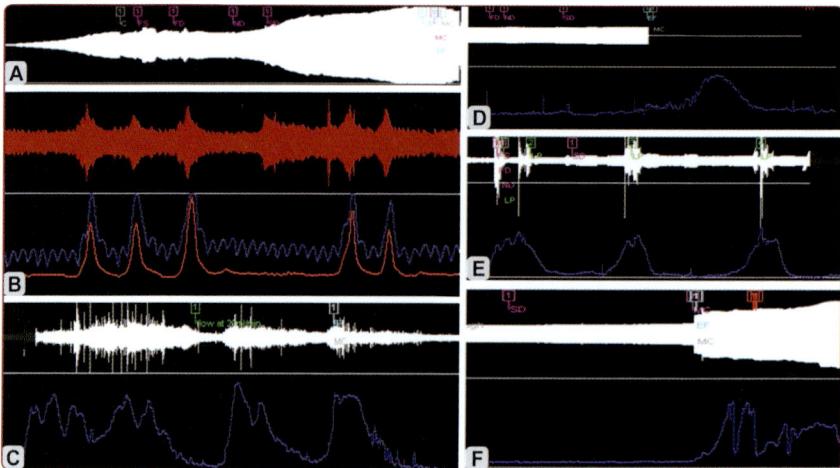

Figs 3A to F: Surface EMG pattern. filling phase: (A) Normal guarding reflex during filling phase—progressively increasing pelvic floor activity with filling; (B) Normal reflex response to cough; (C) Normal reflex response to detrusor overactivity; voiding phase; (D) Normal silence of sphincteric activity during voiding; (E) Detrusor external sphincter dyssynergia; (F) Nonrelaxation of sphincter during voiding in dysfunctional elimination syndrome

report bladder sensations with progressive filling. Even bladder pressures could be measured watching the height of water column. This was a useful, though crude and unstandardized method of evaluating storage function of bladder. There were several limitations:

- The measured bladder pressure (Pves) would not truly represent the detrusor pressure (Pdet), since the Pves would be the sum of Pdet and extravesical abdominal pressure (Pabd)
- Various events, like straining and detrusor overactivity, etc. would not be assessable
- Voiding phase could not be assessed
- Pelvic floor activity could not be assessed.

With improved understanding, and design of equipment and catheters, multichannel cystometry has become standard of care. It has been standardized by International Continence Society and the guidelines published (2002). It consists of the following channels:
a. Vesical pressure (Pves)
b. Abdominal pressure (Pabd)
c. Electromyography (EMG)

Preparation of the Patient

The following must be ensured:
- A sterile urine culture—a single dose of suitable antimicrobial with gram negative coverage should be administered before the test

- Empty rectum—preferably by natural means. Sometimes, in patients with constipation (neurogenic or non-neurogenic), it becomes imperative to use laxatives/purgatives (e.g. picosulfate, enema). Downside of using these agents is involuntary rectal contractions during the test, which would make interpretation of Pdet confounded (Figure 4)
- An informed consent.

Performing the Test

Multichannel urodynamics is not a standalone investigation for complete interpretation of a clinical condition. It often, rather always, requires great amount of feedback from clinical picture and other investigations. The contributing reasons are:
- Bladder filling at supra-normal rates (solution: ambulatory UDS)
- Filling solution (normal saline with or without iodinated contrast) often not at body temperature (solution: using prewarmed solution)
- Changes due to catheterization:
  ➤ Relative narrowing of lumen caliber due to the presence of a catheter
  ➤ Sphincteric spasm and pain
  ➤ Alteration in lie and position of urethra and urethra-vesical relation
- *Solution:* Using the thinnest possible catheter of soft material and gentle technique.

Therefore, it is imperative to have bladder diary and results of free uroflowmetry with post-void residual urine, available while doing the test. It is important to re-emphasize that in the face of artefacts and limitations of data

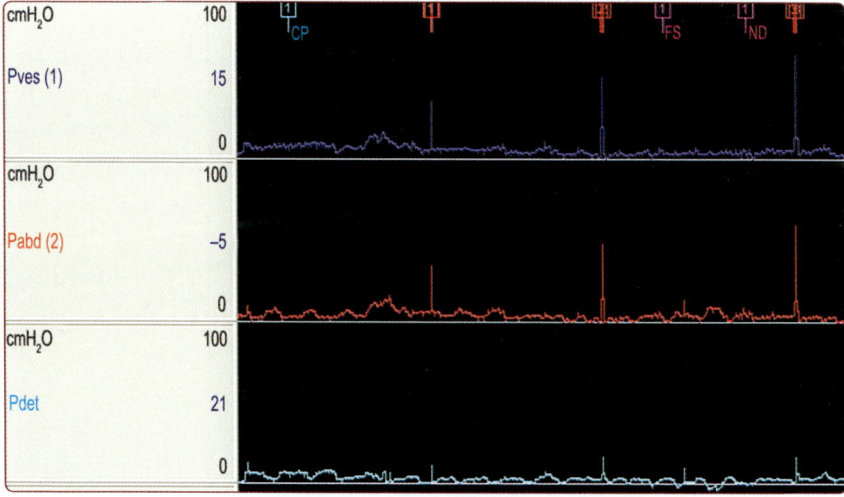

Fig. 4: Involuntary rectal activity (Pabd—red tracing) resulting from purgatives given for preparation for UDS leads to fictitious detrusor overactivity (light blue tracing—bottom line). The relatively silent Pves tracing (topline) compared to Pabd clinches the diagnosis of artifact

acquisition during UDS, the results of UDS must be explainable by the clinical scenario and must not be followed blindly. The interpretation of UDS findings is best done in real-time while performing the test.

Having taken the consent and administering the antibiotic, an effort is made to familiarize the apprehensive patient with the hi-tech surroundings. One can never, and should not, rush through this part of preparation. An apprehensive patient cannot "relax" (the pelvic floor) and "perform" voiding. Once the patient is seated comfortably, the catheters and EMG electrodes are placed. It is convenient to have the patient supine for placement of catheters and then shift on a chair with catheters in situ to be seated for the study. With an electromechanical urodynamic chair, this process is much more convenient both for the urodynamicist as well as the patient, since he/she does not have to shift places (Figures 5A to C). Most of the tests can be performed in the sitting position; occasionally, squatting or standing may be required. Two common scenarios, which would require change in position, are:

❖ Patient with voiding dysfunction not able to pass urine in sitting position: It is not uncommon to misinterpret this situation as "detrusor atonia".

We have found squatting position very useful for helping him/her void without having to strain (straining is as far as avoidable; *vide infra*). In this position, increased intra-abdominal pressure, its transmission to the

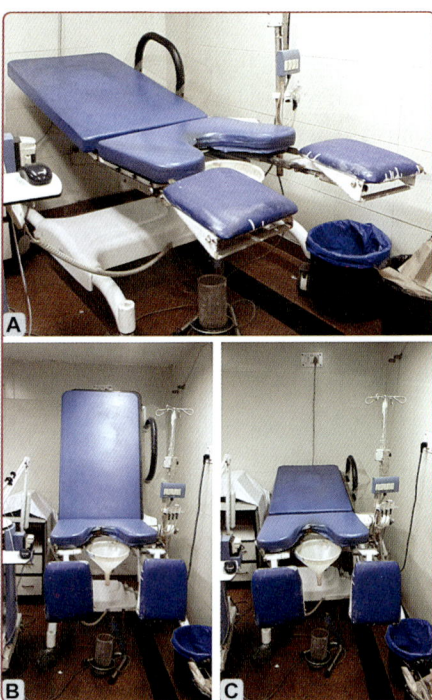

Figs 5A to C: Sonesta fluoroscopic electro-mechanical motorized chair at Urodynamic lab, PGIMER, Chandigarh

bladder, and complete relaxation of anterior and adductor thigh muscles and the pelvic floor can facilitate urinary flow. Having an automated UDS chair is an asset for this position which would not be possible on a simple commode chair. Alternatively, some patients would prefer to void in standing.

❖ Leak not demonstrable in sitting position in a patient with stress urinary incontinence: Squatting or standing position (with thighs spread out) are useful in this scenario.

Since fluid infused catheters are the most commonly used, we will describe this method in the following section:

a. *Fine double lumen cystometry catheter (~6Fr):* One lumen is for the measurement of pressure and the second is for the retrograde filling of bladder. Alternatively, two fine infant feeding tubes (5Fr each) can be inserted; one used for filling and another for pressure measurement. During the voiding phase, the 'infusion tube' can be removed to minimize compromise of urethral lumen. This method is, no doubt, cost effective; however, dislodgement of catheter and unstandarized compliance of the feeding tube material remain as limitations. Whatever catheter, it is preferable to flush out air before insertion.

Troubleshooting

The catheter not going into the bladder

At the outset, it is assumed that the patient does not have a stricture which can explain patient's symptoms. It would be inappropriate to do a UDS in this scenario. Once the stricture is ruled out (by retrograde urethrography or urethral calibration), presence of sphincter spasm or false passage can pose difficulty in catheterization. It can be dealt with by passing a hydrophilic guidewide (≤ 0.032-inch diameter for a 6Fr catheter) and threading the catheter over it. Alternatively, foley can be used as a catheter-guide as follows (Figure 6):

➲ Catheter tip engaged in the eye of a 14Fr foley catheter
➲ The assembly is passed into the bladder
➲ The foley is advanced and the catheter pulled a little to disengage
➲ Foley is gently pulled out.

b. *Single lumen balloon catheter (5–10Fr):* Most commonly for rectal placement (Figure 7); in women, vaginal catheters can be used for this purpose. Rarely, patients on ileostomy/colostomy (most commonly after abdomino-perineal resection), these stomata would be the entry-points for this measurement. It is assumed that any pressure transmission in abdomen (e.g. straining) to the bladder is identical to the rectum or vagina. Alternatively, a glove finger (with small slit) tied on 8Fr infant feeding tube can be made to do the same job. Whatever catheter, it is preferable to flush out air before insertion.

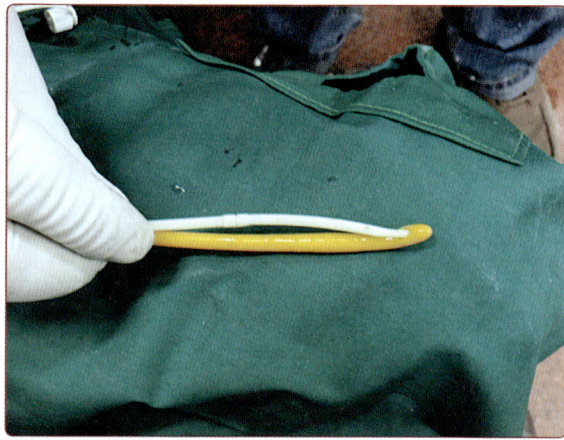

Fig. 6: Method of inserting UDS catheter in case of difficulty, particularly for inserting a stiff catheter. Insert the tip of catheter into the eye of a 14Fr foley catheter and insert the assembly into the urethra

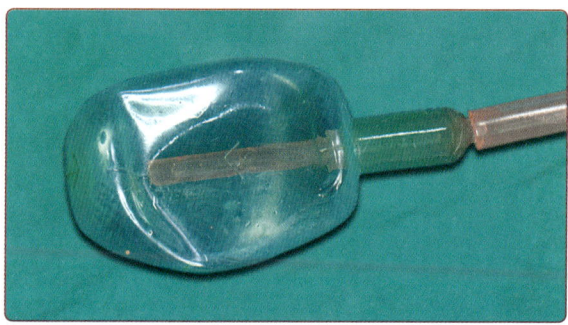

Fig. 7: Single lumen rectal balloon catheter; a small angular slit is visible in the center of the balloon

c. *Electromyography:* Using surface electrodes; two active electrodes on either side of the anus and one neutral electrode not too far from the active electrodes on the buttock or perineum.

Displacement of catheters is not an uncommon happening during UDS, particularly when the patient strains to void or during valsalva maneuver, particularly in women. It is, therefore, important to fix these in position to avoid problems during the test (Figures 8A and B). Naturally, clipping, shaving or depilating cream application for local hair removal would facilitate the fixation.

Catheters and electrodes are connected to the respective transducers. Once the catheters are fixed in position and connected to the transducers, the imperative next step is to free those of air inside the channel, by flushing with infusion fluid. Any amount of air in the system from the syringe to tip of catheter will dampen the recording.

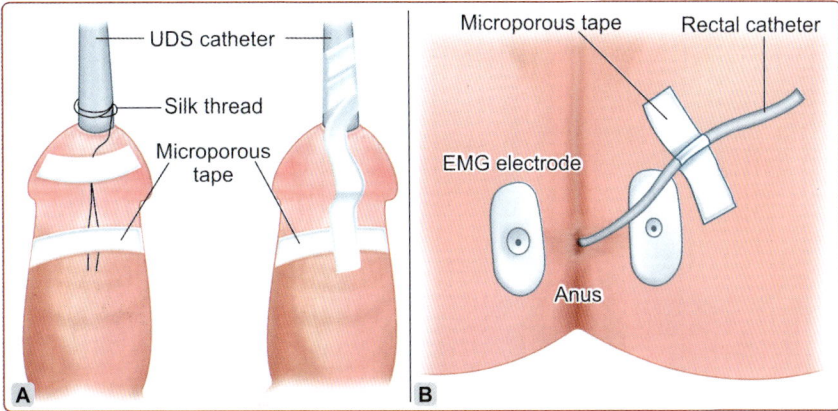

Figs 8A and B: Methods of fixing: (A) Cystometry catheter, and (B) Rectal catheter to avoid slippage. To note, UPP catheter is fixed to the puller and, therefore, does not require fixation to the body

Next, position of catheters and sensitivity of transducers is checked by asking the patient to cough; deflection in vesical and abdominal readings should be equal without a phase difference. This is reflected in nil (or nearly so) deflection in Pdet graph; a small biphasic deflection is acceptable.

> **Troubleshooting**
>
> In case deflection is more than small, or is not biphasic, something is wrong in the connections. One should systematically check the positioning of catheter, flush out any possible air bubble, any kink or knot in the tubing-extension, connection of transducer-dome to the transducer and, lastly, the integrity of transducer, catheter and dome.
>
> Sometimes, in patients with patulous anal tone or fecal impaction, Pabd would not record properly. One can try placing the rectal catheter far inside or try 'plugging' the anus with, say, a foley catheter. In the presence of fecal impaction, it is better to postpone the study till the clearing of bowel.

Zeroing

Once the connections are in order, the next mandatory step is zeroing, i.e. all the transducers are measuring atmospheric pressure (taken as zero) at a given point in relation to the patient's bladder. This point is superior border of pubic symphysis.

The procedure is as follows (Figures 9A to C):
- Both the transducers (Pves and Pabd) are placed at the above-mentioned level.

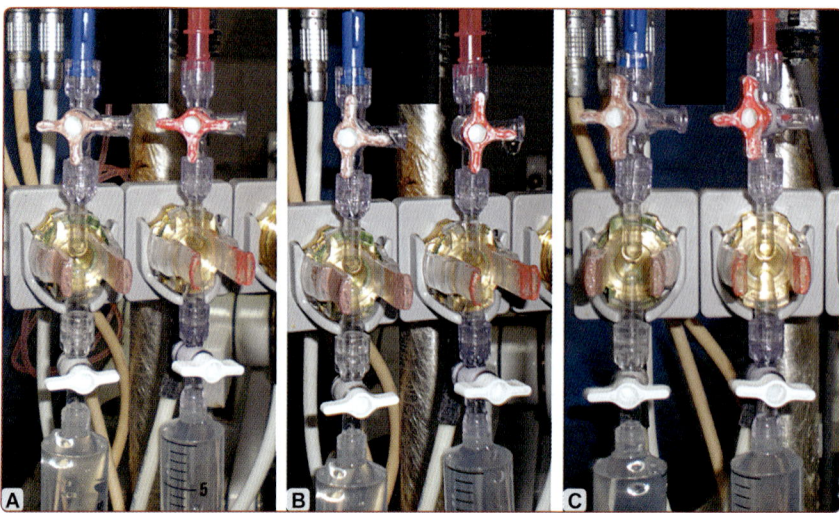

Figs 9A to C: Process of zeroing: (A) Expose the transducers to the atmospheric pressure only (cutting those off from the bladder and rectal pressures) and press zero; (B) Alternatively, the transducers as well as internal pressures can be exposed to the atmospheric pressures before zeroing; (C) after 'zero all', the transducers are cut-off from the atmospheric pressures and exposed only to internal pressures. To note, in all the steps, syringes are cut-off to avoid pressure leak into the syringes

- After flushing the transducers and catheters with saline, the syringe connection is blocked from the transducer by rotating the two-way connector.
- The three-way connections of the transducers are opened to atmosphere, with or without the measurement catheters and the 'zero all' button is pressed. This way all the three lines (Pves, Pabd and Pdet) show 'zero' reading.
- Now, the three-way connector is rotated so that the transducers are connected to the interior and disconnected from the atmosphere. This shows certain reading in Pves and Pabd (supine 10–20 cm H2O; sitting 15–40 cm H2O and standing 30–50 cm H2O)
- The Pdet at this point should show a near-zero value assuming Pves and Pabd are equal and the detrusor activity is zero with empty bladder. Any minor correction can be done by the computer software using "*Pdet to zero*" command.

Basic measurements (channels):
- Total vesical pressure (Pves)
- Abdominal pressure (Pabd)
- Detrusor pressure (Pdet)—this is the true pressure exerted by the elements of bladder wall (detrusor and fibro-elastic tissue). This is an indirect

measurement and is derived (by the software) by subtracting Pabd from Pves on real-time basis
- EMG (to be detailed later)
- Infused volume (Vinf)
- Flow rates (Qura)
- Voided volume (VV).

THE FILLING PHASE

While the patient is in the sitting position, the infusion is started. The initial rate of infusion can be determined as per the following principles:
- Conventionally, the flow rates were classified as slow (upto 10 mL/min.), medium (10–100 mL/min.) and fast (>100 mL/min.). Most commonly, a medium rate was selected—the problem was a wide range
- The current guidelines classify the rate as physiological (upto 25% of body weight) and supra-physiological; the former rate is selected for most cases
- Another convenient way is to initiate inflow at a rate ~10% of bladder capacity, determined by bladder diary. We most often commence at 30 mL/min. in most cases and vary the rate as the study goes on.

In general patients with detrusor overactivity and poor compliance, it is suggested to keep the flow slow to avoid artefacts. On the other hand, sometimes provocation of a detrusor overactivity is required. In this situation, a rapid flow and use of relatively cold saline would be helpful.

As the filling continues, the clinician/technician should keep the patient busy in talking to keep him diverted from apprehension of catheters (Figure 10). Proper connections should be periodically checked during the study by asking the patient to gently cough—this should show equal deflection in Pves and Pabd without any significant deflection in Pdet. The EMG should show a deflection as well.

Various sensations/events should be marked in real-time—first sensation, first desire, normal desire, strong desire, any urgency, any leak or pain. We routinely do not fill much beyond strong desire, since it would not add to the information and may affect the results of the voiding phase, since the patient would be uncomfortable.

Compliance

"It describes the relationships between changes in bladder volume and changes in detrusor pressure."
It is calculated by the following formula:
$$= \Delta \text{ volume}/\Delta \text{ detrusor pressure.}$$

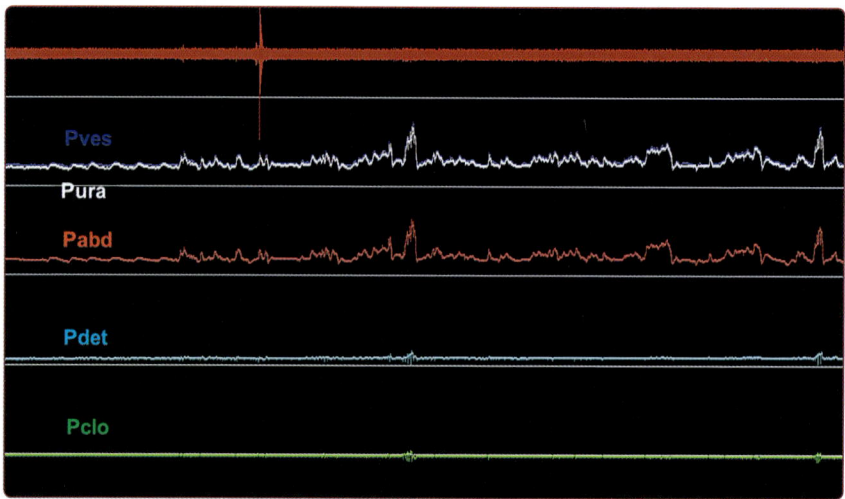

Fig. 10: During filling, the urodynamicist should keep the patient busy in talking to him/her to allay anxiety. In the UDS graph, irregular Pves, Pura and Pabd tracings represent a continuous verbal interaction; silent Pdet (= Pves − Pabd) and Pclo (= Pura − Pves) show immaculate connections without any obstruction or air in tubings

Therefore, the overall compliance of the filling cycle = MCC/end-fill Pdet (assuming initial Pdet to be zero).

MCC = Maximum cystometric capacity

The following caveats should be kept in mind while calculating the compliance:

- In patients with terminal DO, end-filling Pdet should be taken at a point just before the start of the DO
- In patients with phasic DO, the above formula is likely to overestimate compliance, since the effect of the entire DOs during filling will be overlooked. Under these circumstances, some UDS equipment (including our Solar Silver®, MMS) have the facility of "linear regression calculation" of compliance, which would take the entire filling cycle into consideration (Figure 11)
- In patients with poor compliance, it is imperative to assess the contribution of muscular (active) and fibro-collagenous (passive) components. For this, the flow should be stopped for about a minute or so and the trend of Pdet should be monitored
- The findings are interpreted as follows (Figure 12):
  - If it remains stable, the likelihood of contribution of active component is remote and the recorded end-filling Pdet is the true value
  - If it begins to fall, there is significant active component due to slow relaxation of detrusor and one should wait for a couple of minutes and record the new Pdet for compliance calculation. The reason of slow relaxation may be a 'too high' fill rate, occult detrusor overactivity or denervated bladder.

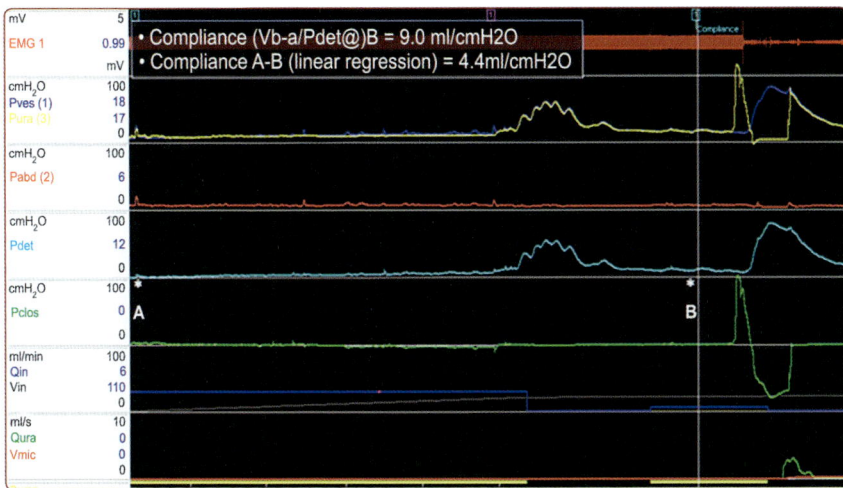

Fig. 11: Comparison of calculation of compliance between simple formula (= cystometric capacity/end-fill Pdet) versus computer-based linear regression in the cases of phasic detrusor overactivity

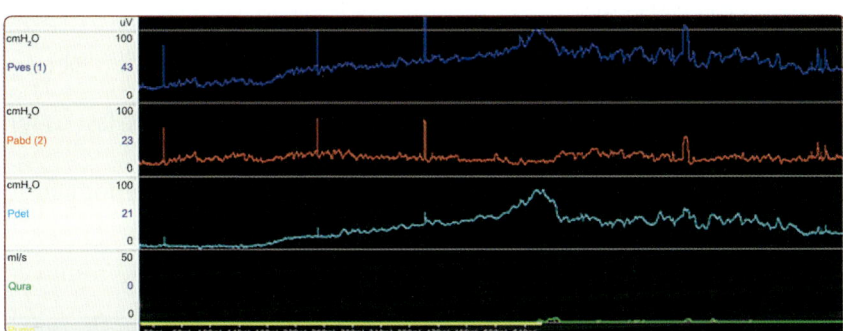

Fig. 12: A patient with prolapse intervertebral disc L5-S1 having lower motor neuron dysfunction type bladder. Poor compliance is evident by progressive steep rise in Pdet with filling. The Pdet at the point of leakage (bottom green tracing) represents detrusor leak-point pressure. Slowly falling Pdet on stopping infusion shows active component (muscular tonus)—this patient was successfully managed with anticholinergics and CIC. Yellow line represents fluid infusion

These findings would also guide the clinician whether or not to consider anticholinergics/botulinum toxin or proceed directly to augmentation cystoplasty (if indicated).

The Leak Point Pressures

a. DLPP (Detrusor Leak Point Pressure): The measurement of DLPP is relevant in patients with poor compliance who are at risk of upper tract deterioration. It is defined as detrusor pressure at which urinary leakage occurs in the absence of any active DO or abdominal straining. A high value (~40 cm H2O; determined by Sir EJ McGuire in children with meningomyelocele) will risk the upper tracts.

b. ALPP (Abdominal Leak Point Pressure): The measurement of ALPP is relevant in the patients with stress urinary incontinence and low values of ALPP are associated with the significant intrinsic sphincter deficiency and with high grade incontinence (<60 cm H2O ISD versus >90 cm H2O urethral hypermobility in women; Sir EJ McGuire). It can be measured by progressive valsalva (e.g. inflating a balloon, straining as if defecating) or progressively intensive cough. At first, it is elicited at 150 mL, if not present, it is again performed at 300 mL. How to demonstrate leak:

a. Fluoroscopy (video-UDS)—highly sensitive.
b. Direct visualization—highly sensitive, preferable by us in view of low cost and most direct evidence.
c. Uroflowmeter—insensitive; only large volume leak will be demonstrated that too with a delay—pressure measurement corroborating with leak will be inaccurate.
d. Stress urethral pressure profilometry—sensitive, not widely studied (detailed later).

In general, CLPP is higher than VLPP for the following reasons (Figure 13):
- Cough initiates a reflex contraction of pelvic muscles
- The true value of CLPP is difficult to identify between Pves at the last cough with no leak, and that with a leak.

Therefore, it is relevant to mention which manoeuvre was performed to elicit ALPP; VLPP is preferable.

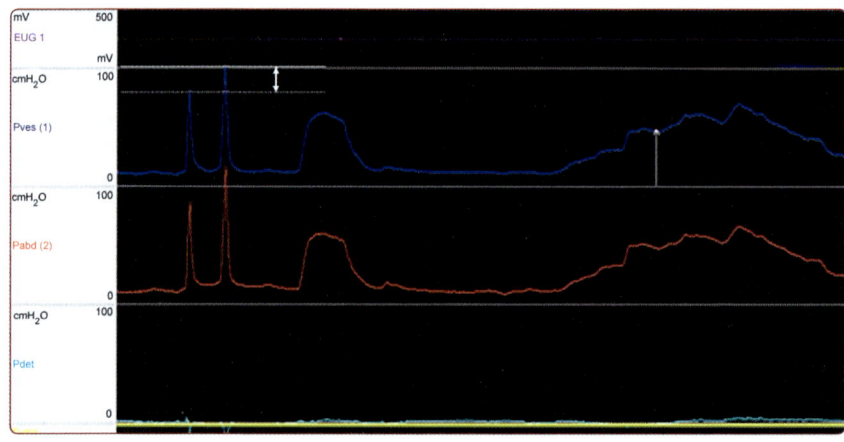

Fig. 13: Graphic representation of cough and valsalva leak point pressures. The difficult interpretation of exact CLPP is shown

Detrusor Overactivity

It is a urodynamic observation characterized by involuntary detrusor contractions during the filling phase, which may be spontaneous or provoked. There is no minimum cut-off of Pdet to define presence of DO; earlier cut-offs of 15 cm H2O have given way. However, generally, a high-quality UDS apparatus is required to reliably detect a DO of amplitude < 5 cm H2O. It can be classified as phasic/sporadic/terminal; or inhibit/uninhibit.

Degree of DO may have implications in outcome of treatment; for example, in patients with mixed incontinence undergoing sling procedures, patients of clinical benign prostatic enlargement with severe LUTS (mixed type) refractory to medical treatment and patients with overactive bladder symptoms. Efforts have been made to quantify the DO, in terms of cumulative average Pdet at DO per unit filling volume as follows:

Detrusor overactivity index (DOI) = $(Pdet_{DO1} + Pdet_{DO2} + Pdet_{DO3}......+Pdet_{DOn})/MCC$

MCC = maximum cystometric capacity

Some machines have software to calculate area under curve (AUC) of recorded parameters (Pves, Pabd, Pura, etc.) [Figure 14]. If it is available, detrusor overactivity index can be calculated as follows:

$$DOI = (AUC_{Pdet} = AUC_{Pves} - AUC_{Pabd})/MCC$$

Despite potential of clinical utility, the DOI remains to be poorly studied, and therefore, not standardized.

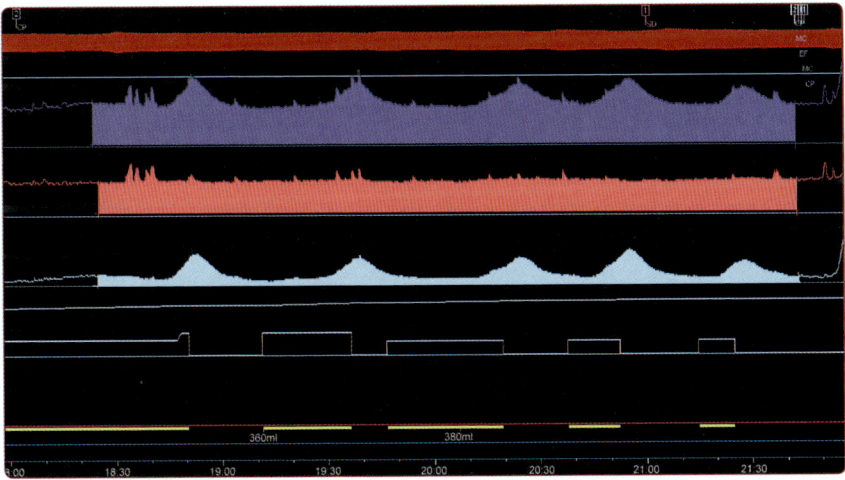

Fig. 14: Graphic representation of calculating area under curve of Pves and Pabd. To note, AUC Pdet is calculated as (AUC Pves − AUC Pabd)

THE MICTURITION PHASE

Most of the time, patient is asked for micturition in the same position as filling, i.e. mostly sitting. Needless to say, the patient should be made calm and relaxed before he/she is asked to pass urine. Complete privacy must be maintained. Patient should be reassured to take his/her own time, and not to strain to perform the void. It is a common tendency to actually do the opposite and end up having non-interpretable results of the voiding phase. It is often helpful to start the tap (for sound of running water) and go out of the patient area to leave him/her alone, and use remote control for markings. Sometimes, however, despite care, he or she may not generate detrusor pressure to void. It is worthwhile, changing the posture to standing or squatting position for trial of voiding. In our experience, many patients have voided successfully in the latter position, failing attempt in sitting or standing position. The physiology behind this position—related phenomenon is multifactorial. Squatting position leads to relaxation of adductor and quadriceps muscles of thigh. This, in turn, helps relaxation of pelvic floor muscles, and the inhibitory effect on detrusor contraction is released. Additionally, abdominal pressure rises in squatting position further facilitating the act of voiding.

Once the micturition is successfully initiated, the patient should be repeatedly encouraged to keep on relaxing while voiding, and that they are doing well. Care should be taken so that all micturate falls in the funnel and not outside; any urine falling outside will not be recorded by the flowmeter and resulting in erroneous pressure-flow relations. Upon completion of the void, bladder should be manually emptied to note exact amount of the post-void residual urine. This helps in minimizing computer's calculation error (PVR = MCC – VV) due to urine production during the study. Typically, once the 'end study' command is given, a 'measure PVR' window appears (this function may not be available in some machines); at this time, the residual should be emptied into the flowmeter. The difference in measured PVR and calculated PVR gives the amount of urine produced during the study. Sometimes, the difference is large enough to change the calculation of compliance (MCC/Pdet) and voiding efficiency (100 – %PVR). Typically, the following parameters are recorded in the micturition phase:

a. Opening Pdet—pressure at which the flow starts.
b. Pdet at Qmax—detrusor pressure corresponding to Qmax.
c. Pdet max—maximum detrusor pressure.
d. Flow rate—average (Qave), maximum (Qmax).
e. Flow time—time to Qmax, flow time.
f. Post-void residue—calculated (MCC – VV), measured (bladder emptied into flow-meter) vide supra.

Tip

It should be emphasized that there is an inevitable lag between recording of pressure and flow, which corresponds to the time taken by the fluid to reach the flow meter jar (typically less than 1 sec). This must be taken into account when measuring pressure-flow relation. This lag can be adjusted for, during calibration process of the UDS machine.

Once the study is completed, one should record a cough to insure equal sensitivity (or any difference thereof) at the end of the study. Although, it will not make any difference in the recorded data, it may help in interpretation (Figures 15A and B). This is particularly of importance, when patient has voided with abdominal straining; a discrepant recording of Pves and Pabd may give a false impression of detrusor contraction, while it may have been absent.

We prefer to repeat the whole study after completion. We believe that it minimizes the artifactual abnormalities aroused out of patient's adjustment problems with catheters and cold artificial infusion.

Interpretation of the Results

Before interpretation of voiding phase, we must understand that bladder has its own properties independent of urethra. Similarly, urethra has its own properties independent of bladder. Nevertheless, both are as much interlinked. To understand further, the author has elaborated concepts of bladder output relations (BOR) and urethral resistance relations (URR).

Bladder contraction is the source of energy for a flow to occur. It is the urethral resistance, which determines how efficiently this energy will be used as kinetic energy in the form of flow (Q) and the rest to remain as static form (Pdet). Therefore, urethral resistance splits the bladder contraction energy into Pdet and Q, this is known as bladder-output relation (Figures 16A and B). Griffith and colleagues defined detrusor contraction strength in terms of watt factor (mechanical power per unit area of bladder surface) as given below:

$$WF\ (W/m^2) = [(Pdet + a)(Vdet + b) - ab]\ 2\pi$$

$$Vdet = Q/2[3(V + Vo)/4\pi]^{2/3}.$$

Here, a = 25 cm H2O, b = 6 mL/s, and Vo = 10 mL.

Pdet during flow is not a direct measure of detrusor strength; it is the pressure when flow stops (Pdet.iso), which is a direct measure of detrusor strength. Since calculation of WF is very complex, an approximation has been made [Pdet.iso ≈ 10 x WF]. In presence of increased urethral resistance, Pdet is increased which is often misinterpreted as 'increased detrusor strength'. It is to be noted that actually detrusor strength, if at all, only decreases with continued obstruction when detrusor tends to give way to resistance. The numerical value

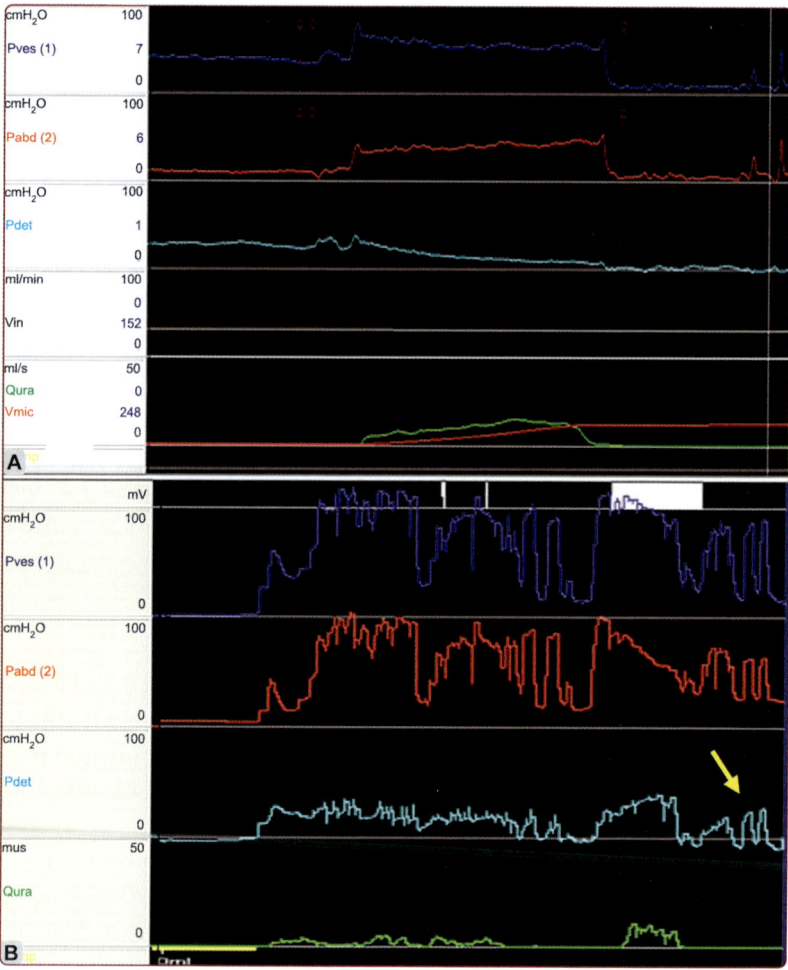

Figs 15A and B: (A) Pressure flow study in a patient with orthotopic neobladder showing perfect cough response at the end of the study. The study is clearly demonstrating voiding entirely by abdominal effort with inactive detrusor contraction. The gradually decreasing Pdet with voiding indicates decreasing passive pressure with emptying; (B) Pressure flow study in a patient with prolapsed intervertebral disc. The cough response at the end of the study is discrepant evident by Pdet peaks (solid arrow). This explains 'apparent active Pdet', during the study, exactly corresponding to each episode of straining. The correct interpretation is non-contraction of detrusor

of Pdet is the outcome of less release of detrusor energy into kinetic energy of flow coupled with decreased compliance.

Flow in rigid tube is directly proportional to cross-sectional area, in the presence of constant pressure (Q α A). The flow starts as soon as there is any pressure upstream. Urethra is a collapsible dynamic elastic tube (and not a rigid one, as used to be once); therefore, some of the bladder's energy would

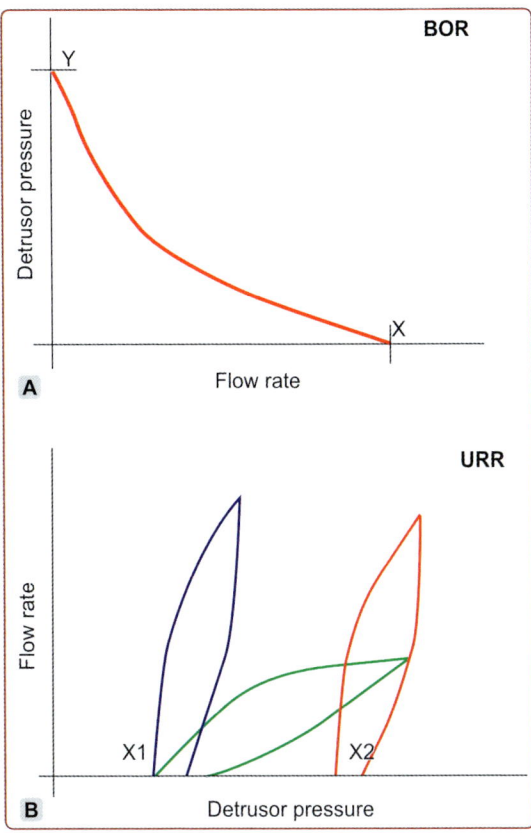

Figs 16A and B: (A) Bladder output relations. Point X is the maximum possible Pdet (equivalent to Pdet iso) and Y is a theoretical point indicating maximum possible flow rate if resistance is tending to zero. BOR is volume specific. (B) Urethral resistance relation—blue line indicates a normal curve, green line a constrictive obstruction (e.g. stricture) and red line a compressive obstruction (e.g. prostatic enlargement). X1 and X2 indicate Pmuo—in constrictive obstruction, Pmuo does not change, whereas, in compressive obstruction, Pmuo increases. Therefore, there are higher chances of retention in the latter type of obstruction

be consumed in overcoming the elastic resistance of urethra before the flow is initiated (opening Pdet). Once the flow is initiated, flow rapidly increases with small increase in pressure. At some point, the flow controlling zone of urethra opens maximally (giving the Pdet Qmax-Qmax point) after which again the behavior changes and flow stops, once the passive urethral elasticity overcomes prevailing detrusor contraction (Pclo); a pressure which is just enough to maintain urethra in open position toward the end of micturition is called as Pmuo (Figures 16A and B). This is a very important concept validated in prostatic obstruction and is roughly equal to the AG number. Derivation of its numerical value is detailed below in Schafer nomogram section.

To summarize, status of bladder contractility and presence or absence of bladder outlet obstruction should be reported separately, as under:

1. *Detrusor contraction strength:* It is quantified by isovolumetric detrusor contraction (Pdet iso) as discussed above. Since this Pdet iso is volume dependent, Griffiths and Schafer conceptualized projected isovolumetric contraction (PIP) as a measure of the above. In males with BPH, this PIP is termed as detrusor contractility index (DCI) as per the following equation:

   $DCI = Pdet.Qmax + (5 \times Qmax)$

   Its reference values in this population are as under:
   - <50—very weak
   - 50–100—weak
   - 100–150—normal
   - >150—strong

   In females with urgency incontinence, PIP was defined as [Pdet Qmax + Qmax]; its normal range was considered to be 30–75.

2. *Bladder outlet obstruction:* Several authors have made phenomenal attempts to numerically define presence of BOO in males and females. Conceptually, the following parameters are measures of degree of BOO, and both are independently important in their own way:

   a. *Pmuo:* As discussed earlier, it is the detrusor pressure required to maintain urethra in open condition towards the end of the void. Therefore, it is somewhat related to closure pressure ($Pdet_{clo}$). It must be emphasized that it is not the same as opening pressure ($Pdet_{open}$). In a given pressure-flow recording, it roughly corresponds to Pdet value, just before the trailing part of uroflow (last 5–10 mL; with Q < 2 mL/s); this trailing is considered to be coming from emptying of urethra, when the outlet has actually closed. Pmuo can be derived from the following equation:

   $Pmuo \approx 40 \times OCO$

   Where, OCO (obstruction coefficient) = $PdetQmax/[40 + (2 \times Qmax)]$.

   Typically, it is at an increased level in patients with prostatic enlargement and bladder neck obstruction; whereas, in patients with stricture urethra, it remains within the normal range.

   b. *Curvature of pressure-flow relation:* Actual curve is a complex one and therefore, not categorizable into one type (Figures 17A and B). Therefore, investigators have derived linear and quadratic simplifications for an approximation with reasonable accuracy.

   PQ_{slope} linear = $(PdetQmax - Pmuo)/Qmax$
   PQ_{slope} quadratic = $(PdetQmax - Pmuo)/Qmax^2$

   The latter is more universally acceptable in keeping with the elastic collapsible tube model of urethra. Passive urethral resistance relation

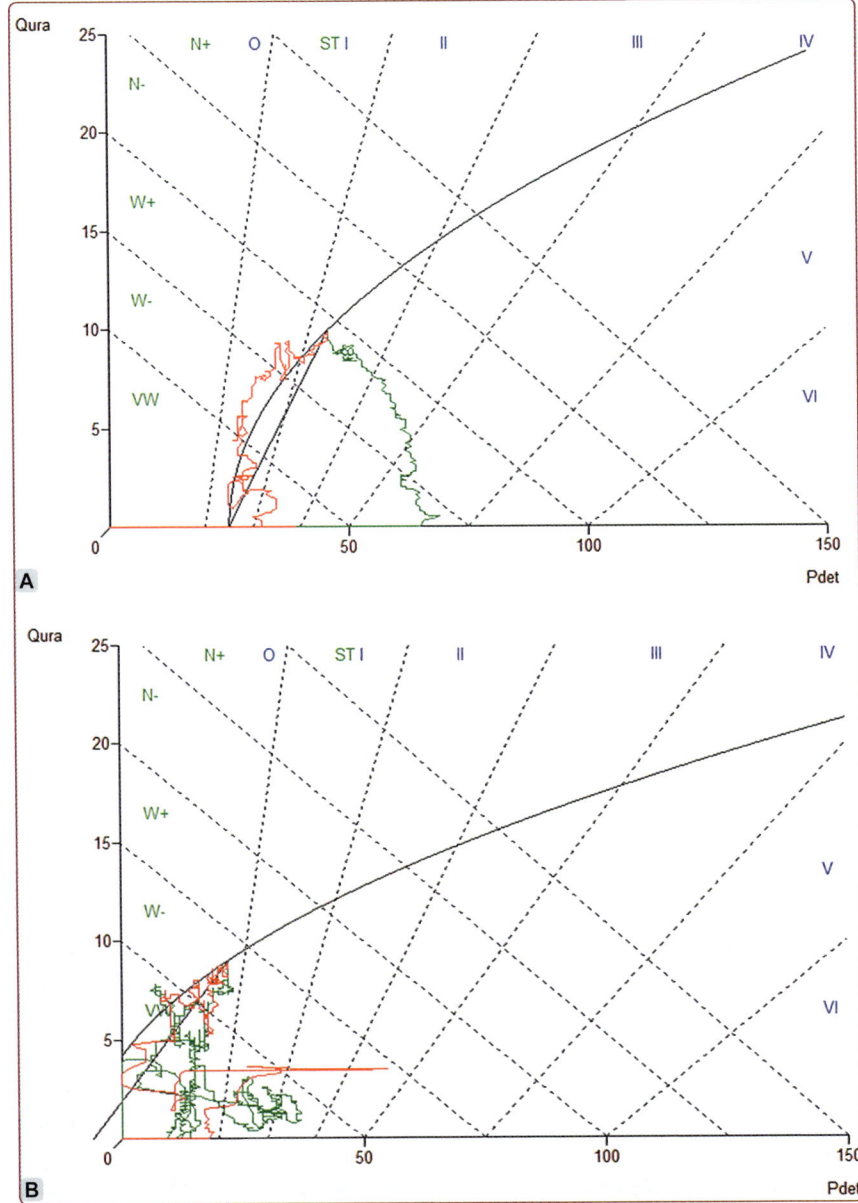

Figs 17A and B: Actual pressure-flow curve (A) A relatively straightforward curve; (B) A complex curve difficult to fit into any pattern—approximations must be made

(PURR) takes into account both these parameters, and is independent of detrusor contraction strength and volume.

Several authors have done phenomenal work to unfold the enigma of pressure-flow relations, and be able to represent it numerically and graphically. Some prominent works are described as under:

i. *Abrams-griffiths nomogram (Figure 18):* They proposed AG number as a measure of BOO, as per the following equation:
AG (or BOO index) = PdetQmax − (2 × Qmax)
Reference values:
- <15 : unobstructed
- 15–40 : equivocal (later modified as 20–40 by International Continence Society Working Committee)
- >40 : obstructed

It must be emphasized that the investigators derived the above concept of AG nomograms and AG number in patients with normal to strong detrusor contractility. It can be understood that in presence of weak detrusor, the numerical value of AG>40 may not be reached. In these equivocal cases, they suggested to look for values of Pmuo and linear slope of pressure-flow relation [PQ_{slope} = (PdetQmax − Pmuo)/Qmax]. Pmuo> 40 cm H2O or PQ_{slope}> 2 cm H2O/mL suggests BOO.

ii. *Schafer nomogram (Figure 19):* Schafer presented detrusor contractility and degree of BOO on one graph, eponymed as *Schafer nomogram*. Detrusor contractility lines were drawn based on equation of DCI (*vide supra*) and contractility was classified into very weak (VW), through W(- and +), normal (N- and +) to strong (ST). Line between W+ and N- represented DCI of 100.

Pressure-flow relation lines were based on the concept of obstruction coefficient (OCO):
OCO = PdetQmax/[40 + (2 × Qmax)].
Progressively increasing degree of obstruction was depicted in 7 grades from 0 to VI. BOO was defined as the presence of >grade II obstruction

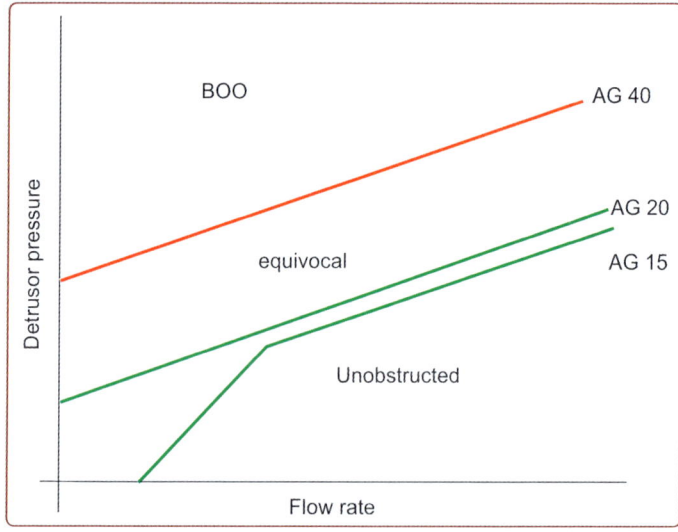

Fig. 18: The Abrams-Griffiths nomogram

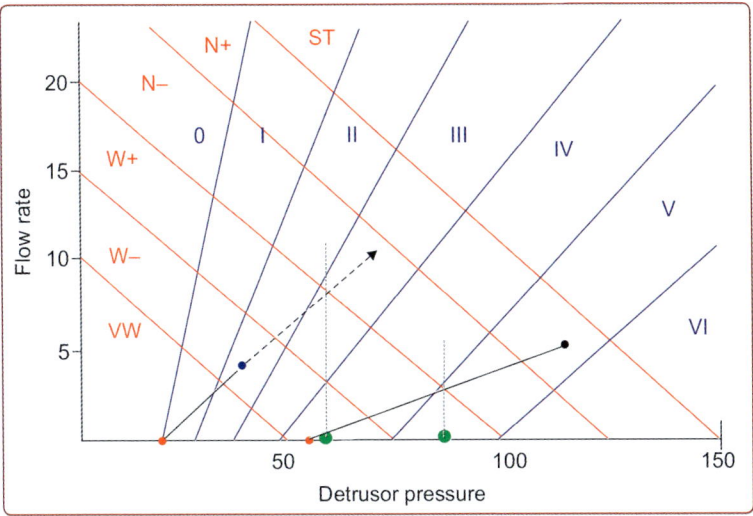

Fig. 19: Schafer nomogram: The location of PdetQmax—Qmax point on the graph represents the status of detrusor contractility as well as bladder outlet obstruction—two PQ relations are drawn. The ascending (blue) lines demarcate degree of BOO (0–VI) and descending (red) demarcate status of detrusor contractility (VW–ST). To calculate DAMPF two points are plotted on the graph—(red dot) Pmuo = 40 x OCO (see text), (blue dot) PdetQmax-Qmax point. Draw a vertical line from the intersection of the line joining these two points and detrusor contractility line between W+ and N-; the point at which this vertical line crosses X axis is DAMPF (green dot).

and equivocal as between grade I–II. To improve sensitivity of diagnosis of BOO in presence of weak detrusor, he conceptualized detrusor-adjusted mean PURR (passive urethral resistance relation) factor [DAMPF] which would represent Pdet iso under standardized conditions of DCI of 100. Unfortunately, he did not come out with validated cut-off values dissimilar to AG number. Calculation of DAMPF is discussed in Figure 18.

iii. *CHESS plot:* In the earlier discussion of BOR and URR, it was evident that apart from higher Pmuo, the curve of BPH was similar to normal individual; whereas, in stricture Pmuo, remained within normal range but the curvature was steeper. With experience, we have found that pressure-flow of patients with external sphincter dysfunction behave similar to constrictive pattern.

Hofner, et al found that Pmuo and curvature were mutually independent parameters of BOO. Therefore, keeping in mind a more accurate diagnosis and characterization of BOO, they conceptualized this two-dimensional plot (Figure 20). This checkerboard-like graph utilizes two independent measures of BOO, i.e. Pmuo (Pvoid min) and quadratic curvature of pressure-flow plot. The curvature is calculated as per the following equation:

Curvature (C) = $(PdetQmax - Pmuo)/Qmax^2$

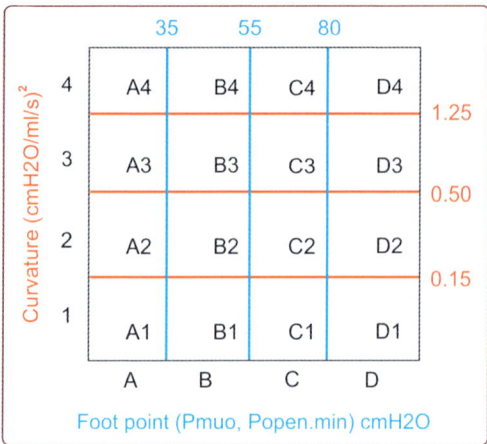

Fig. 20: CHESS 2-dimensional plot

Cell A1 signifies absence of BOO (the patient may have normal, weak or strong detrusor contractility), A4 perfect stricture (or EUS dysfunction as we have found), D1 perfect BPH and D4 perfect bladder neck obstruction.

Defining BOO in women

The voiding physiology is quite different in women from men. Due to low urethral resistance, they void with much lower Pdet. In fact, upto a third of normal would void without any appreciable rise in Pdet, with some abdominal straining only. There is no standardized criteria for diagnosis of BOO in women. Initially, Messy and Abrams recommended presence of 2 or more of the following criteria for diagnosis of BOO:
- Detrusor pressure >50 cm H2O
- Peak flow rate <12 cm H2O
- Urethral resistance factor (=Pdet/Qmax^2) > 0.2
- High PVR in presence of high pressure or resistance factor.

Later, Blaivas and Groutz developed detrusor pressure—free uroflow nomogram and divided female voiding into 4 zones (no, mild, moderate, severe obstruction) [Figure 21]. Lines demarcating mild/moderate and moderate/severe obstruction are horizontal, which means irrespective to flow rate, Pdet max decides level of obstruction (~60 cm H2O and ~110 cm H2O, respectively). Pressure-flow relation is mainly useful in borderline situations, i.e. differentiating normal from mild obstruction.

Detrusor Contraction Pattern

Detrusor contraction pattern has not been described to be of any diagnostic importance. However, in our recent study, we observed a plateau pattern of detrusor contraction (unlike a usual bell-shaped curve) in patients who were

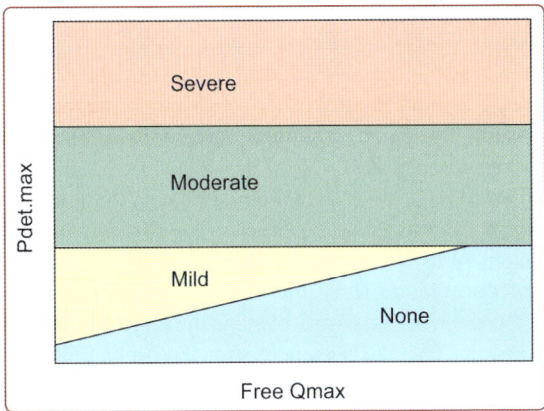

Fig. 21: Blaivas-Groutz nomogram

diagnosed with dysfunction of EUS. Based on scientific explanation and observation of patients with voluntary detrusor contraction, we believe that this phenomenon is secondary to urethra to bladder guarding reflex which persists into voiding phase. Commonly, these patients have high-resting MUCP [Figure 22].

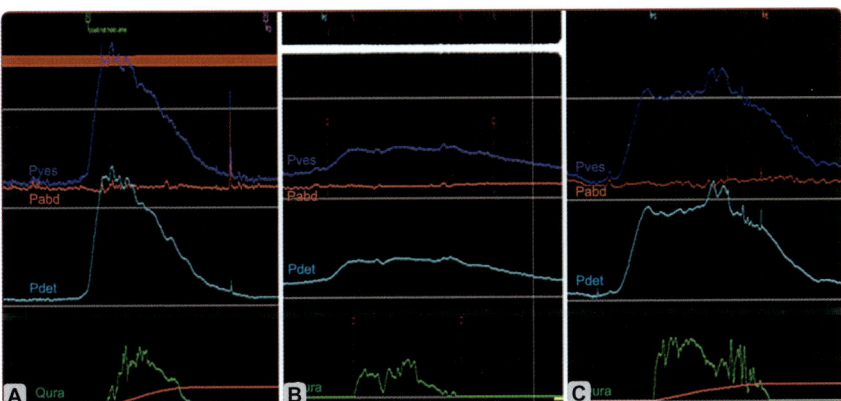

Figs 22A to C: Description of plateau detrusor contraction pattern. (A) Pressure-flow study of a 76-year-old male with benign prostatic enlargement showing typical high pressure-low flow pattern with asymmetrical bell-shaped detrusor pattern (for reference); (B) Pressure-flow study of a 40-year-old male with dysfunctional-elimination syndrome showing low pressure-low flow pattern with plateau detrusor pattern; (C) Pressure-flow study of a 36-year-old male with primary bladder neck obstruction showing high pressure-low flow pattern with plateau at the peak corresponding with voluntary squeeze due to pain during voiding

SUGGESTED READING

1. Agarwal MM, Kamal H, Mavuduru RM. Is it essential to cut-off catheters from transducers while zeroing to atmospheric pressure in preparing for multichannel urodynamic study. Presented at annual conference of North zone chapter of Urological Society of India; 2011.
2. Good Urodynamic Practices: Uroflowmetry, Filling Cystometry and Pressure-Flow Studies Schäfer W, Abrams P, Liao L, et al. NeurourolUrodynam. 2002;21:261–74.
3. Hofner K, Kramer AEJL, Tan K, Krah H, Jonas U. CHESS classification of bladder-outflow obstruction. World J. Urol. 1995;13:59–64.
4. McKinney TB, Goldstein H, Hessami S. comparison of fiberoptic, microtip, water and air-charged pressure transducer catheters for the evaluation of urethral pressure profiles. (Presented at the International Uro-Gynecology Association Meeting, October 2000, Rome Italy).

CHAPTER 5

Video Urodynamics

Functional urethra is the part of urethra which maintains continence. The same urethra is flow controlling zone during voiding process. In males, preprostatic, prostatic and membranous urethra, encompassing internal urethral sphincter, prostate and external sphincter, respectively forms functional urethra. In females, the whole urethra acts as functional urethra and flow controlling zone. Therefore, dysfunction of any of the zones of urethra can lead to bladder outlet obstruction. Diagnosis of BOO using numerical parameters or graphical impressions of pressure-flow study is not a perfect one leaving a grey zone called borderline.

There are several causes of obstruction of functional urethra, bladder neck obstruction (primary or dyssynergia), extrinsic sphincter dysfunction (functional, non-relaxation, dyssynergia, bradykinesia), prostatic obstruction and stricture/stenosis (females). Only in older patients without neurological impairment (e.g. diabetic neuropathy, Parkinsonism, prolapsed intervertebral disk, etc.) presenting with voiding symptoms with clinical prostatic enlargement, it can be assumed with fair certainty that prostate is the cause of obstruction. In all other groups, it is imperative to pinpoint the site and etiology of obstruction, particularly before planning an invasive treatment.

Therefore, there is scope of gathering more information directly from the functional urethra, to supplement the diagnosis, as well as for localization of BOO. There are two methods to achieve the same:
a. Cystourethrography, the anatomical method.
b. Urethral pressure profilometry, the functional method.

Video urodynamics (VUDS) is a combined anatomical and functional study of lower urinary tract. It is essentially performing a dynamic voiding cystourethrography (VCUG) synchronized with pressure-flow study (Figures 1A to C).

SETUP

Quite naturally, the setup for a VUDS is much more elaborate and costly than that of UDS. The first requirement is a bigger room; a 30 sq m room is optimal for VUDS, compared to 20 sq m for UDS without fluoroscopy. The following additional requirements are (Figures 2A and B):
a. A mobile fluoroscopy C-arm machine with height and position adjustable.

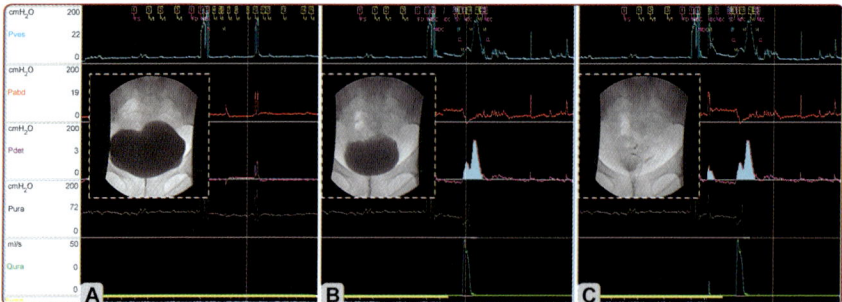

Figs 1A to C: A demo-video of urodynamic study uploaded in MMS software at PGIMER, Chandigarh. Cine fluoroscopy was recorded synchronized with the UDS in filling, (A) Voiding; (B) Postvoid; (C) At the end of the study, as the curser (vertical white line on UDS tracing) is moved forward and backward, fluoro image taken at that moment is displayed

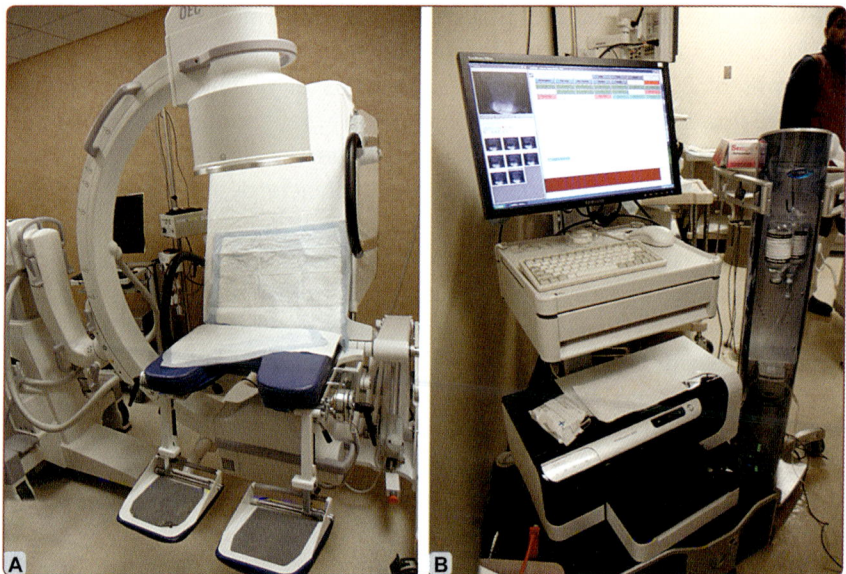

Figs 2A and B: Video urodynamic setup of urology service, Memorial Sloan-Kettering Cancer Center, New York, NY, USA. (A) C-arm fluoroscopy unit placed on video UDS chair (Sonesta); (B) Laborie VUDS system. (courtesy – Dr. Jaspreet Sandhu, Attending Urologist, MSKCC)

b. *An X-ray-compatible urodynamic chair:* Cost of this accessory can be avoided by performing VUDS in standing position or making patient sit on a customized plastic stool with a cut made for urination. However, patient's comfort and convenience of clinician will have to be compromised to some extent.

c. *Hardware and software for integration of fluoroscopy output into UDS:* This cost may be avoided by performing simultaneous fluoroscopy without integration or performing dynamic VCUG on a separate occasion in radiology suite. However, the advantage of real-time synchronization with pressure-flow tracings will be lost.

Nevertheless, clinically useful results are still obtainable. In fact, if done on a separate occasion, a catheterless VCUG may provide potential opportunity for more representative results. At our center, due to financial constraint, we do not have a C-arm in UDS suite. Our high power radio fluoroscopy suite is installed just next door to UDS suite. We, therefore, perform UDS without video and shift the patient to radiology suite immediately for VCUG, if need arises. In our study of 82 patients with voiding dysfunction (under review for publication), we compared outcome of PFS, micturitional UPP and catheterless VCUG done on separate occasions, interpretation of MUPP and VCUG was concordant in all but one patient.

d. An iodinated contrast agent is required for preparing solution for instillation.

Since this is not to be infused intravenously, we use high osmolality contrast material (HOCM) only, typically sodium meglumine diatriazoate (76%). Proprietary iodinated solutions are also available, e.g. cysto-conray^{tm} II (iothalamate meglumine 17.2%, covidien, hazelwood, USA).

PROCEDURE

- We typically prepare 30% contrast solution in 0.9% (w/v) sterile normal saline (i.e. dissolve 76% contrast solution in the NS, in a ratio of 2:5). The contrast agent should not be diluted too much, else urethral anatomy and function would not be appreciable well.
- The uroflowmeter is calibrated with the contrast solution. To note, the specific gravity of this solution is significantly higher than that of NS; therefore, in absence of calibration, a false high reading will be registered by the uroflowmeter. *It feels heavier to catch a solid metal ball than a solid rubber ball of the same size!*
- UDS is performed in the usual manner and fluoroscopy done periodically during filling phase. Typically, X-ray intends on the bladder perpendicularly in AP direction. If reflux is suspected, oblique views are taken to visualize low grade reflux, if present.
- It is imperative to take oblique views in voiding phase. It is very common to miss status of bladder neck in males and the whole urethra in females, if only AP views are taken, severely jeopardizing the benefit of this painstaking, expensive and potentially hazardous (radiation) study [Figures 3(A and B) and 4(A and B)].

INDICATIONS OF VIDEO URODYNAMICS

Virtually, every patient requiring UDS is potentially a candidate of VUDS. This is true, particularly when the problem is anticipated in the bladder outlet (functional urethra). Additional advantage of VUDS (or VCUG) is to detect

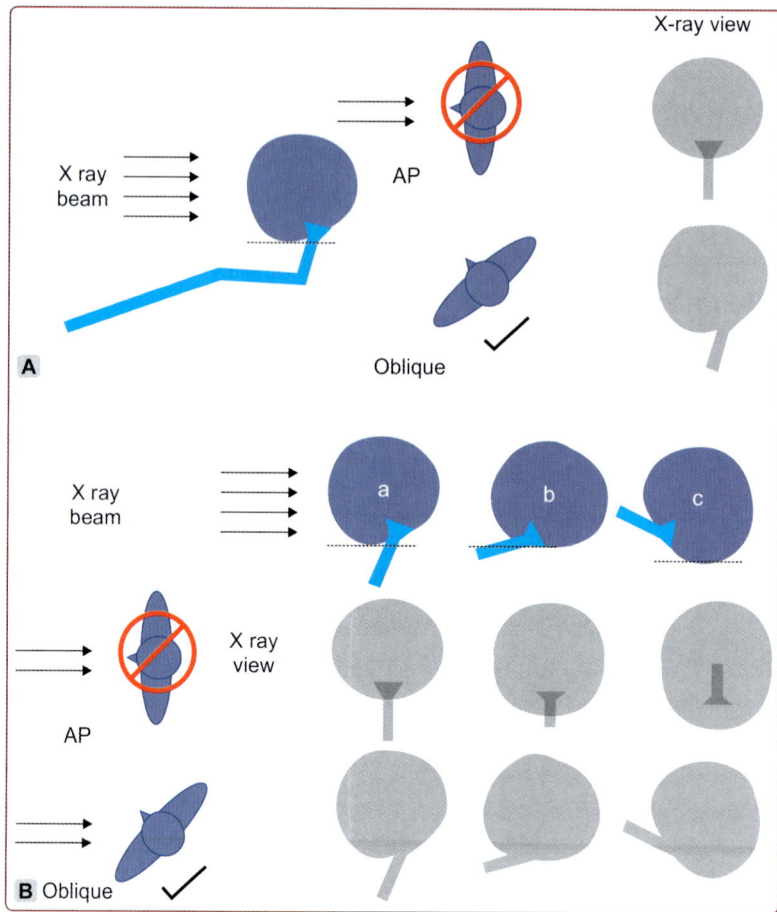

Figs 3A and B: Importance of correct positioning of male (A) and female (B) patient during voiding VUDS or VCUG. (a), (b) and (c) represent normal, mild and severe defect in anterior pelvic support (cystocele), respectively in females. Study done in AP position leads to superimposition of pre-prostatic urethra in male and most or all of urethra in female depending on status of pelvic support and urethral mobility. To note, the best visualization of the functional urethra would be seen in full lateral position (in relation to direction of X-rays). However, due to superimposition of pelvic bones and joints, at good tread-off is at ~450 oblique position

anatomical abnormalities in bladder/functional urethra, which may confound UDS findings, e.g. vesicoureteric reflux, bladder diverticulum, false passage in urethra, etc. Some specific indications of VUDS are as under:

Postprostatectomy Dysfunction

1. *Persistent obstructive symptoms*—Having ruled out a stricture by urethral calibration/retrograde urethrography persistent obstructive symptoms might

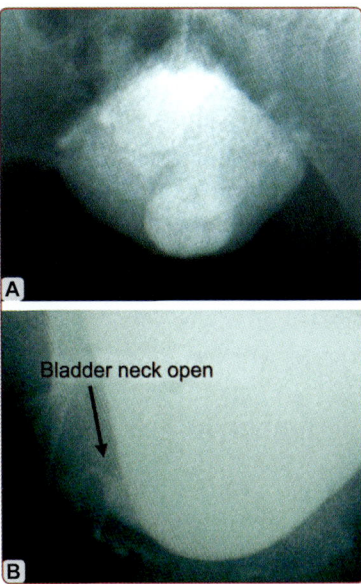

Figs 4A and B: (A) VCUG in a patient with voiding dysfunction done in AP view. urethra completely overlapped by bladder. (B) VCUG repeated in the same patient in oblique view clearly demonstrating widely open bladder neck with non-relaxing EUS

be present for various causes, e.g. detrusor underactivity, residual adenoma or pelvic floor dysfunction. A VUDS is highly informative; micturitional UPP is an excellent alternative.

2. *Incontinence*—It is important to differentiate between urge and stress incontinence; clinical history, examination and bladder diary are very useful. Sometimes, both type of incontinence are present. VUDS helps in differentiating pure DO-related, stress-induced DO-related and pure stress-related incontinence. Leak point pressures can be accurately recorded; although the validity of ALPP in male incontinence has been questioned (ref:). Since male urethra is very long, watching fluid drop at the meatus is too insensitive a method.

Neurogenic Bladder

1. *Integrity of bladder neck*—Meningomyelocele, prolapsed intervertebral lumbar disk. Bladder neck may be incompetent.
2. *Function of bladder neck*—High spinal lesions (above T6) may have bladder neck dyssynergia in addition to external sphincter dyssynergia.
3. *Integrity of external sphincter*—Meningomyelocele, prolapsed intervertebral lumbar disk. Fixed sphincter deformity may be there.

4. *Functions of external sphincter:*
   - Meningomyelocoele, prolapsed intervertebral lumbar disk—fixed sphincter deformity
   - Suprasacral spinal lesions—detrusor sphincter dyssynergia
   - Parkinsonism—sphincter bradykinesia.

Detrusor Underactivity

To differentiate between the primary detrusor underactivity and the pelvic floor dysfunction, we have seen in the previous chapter that a plateau-type detrusor pattern corroborates with the pelvic floor dysfunction.

Stress Urinary Incontinence in Women

1. VUDS is considered to be one of the most sensitive methods to detect leakage; it would detect leakage into the urethra, even before fluid drop comes out of the meatus. Synchronized pressure recording would give an accurate measurement of ALPP.
2. *Urethral hypermobility:* Urethral angle can be accurately calculated by post-processing the image in which the women had a leak during stress maneuver.

To Differentiate Primary Bladder-Neck Obstruction from the Pelvic Floor Dysfunction

Inasmuch as the diagnosis of bladder outlet obstruction, it is imperative to pinpoint the location of obstruction for a targeted therapy. For example, a young man with voiding dysfunction may be suffering from pelvic floor dysfunction rather than bladder neck obstruction. Bladder neck incision without pinpoint diagnosis will not only be ineffective, but also preclude his chances of improvement by any intervention on EUS (for the fear of incontinence). A notable exception to this pinpoint diagnosis may be older man presenting with typical voiding-type of LUTS with clinical enlargement of prostate and a normal neurological history and examination.

ADVANTAGES OF VUDS (OR VCUG DONE SEPARATELY WITHIN A SHORT INTERVAL)

1. May help in detecting anatomical abnormalities likely to be missed in other investigations—these may or may not have immediate clinical implications (Figures 5A to G)
2. Definitive pinpointing of location of obstruction or rule out obstruction, if correlated clinically [Figures 6(A to F) and 7(A to F)].

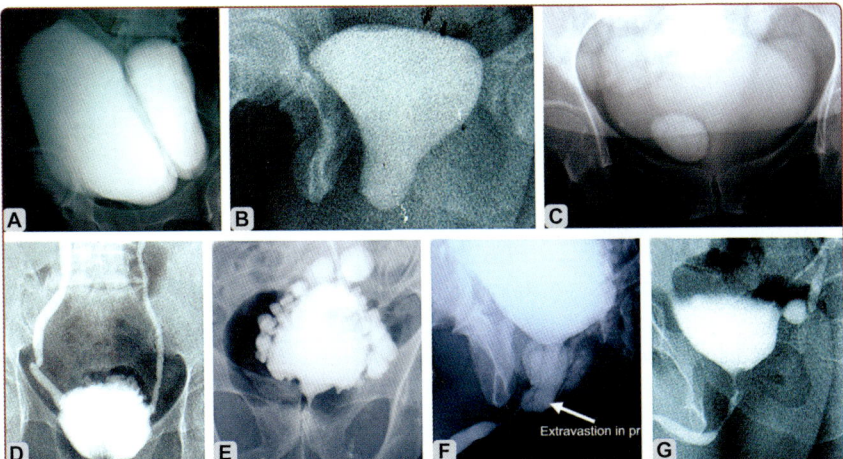

Figs 5A to G: Some abnormalities detected on VCUG performed for voiding dysfunction. (A) Large bladder diverticulum; (B) Stage III cystocele; (C) Calculus within ureterocele; (D) Bilateral vesicoureteral reflux with trabeculated bladder; (E) Diverticulated bladder—status post prostatectomy; (F) Intraprostatic reflux; (G) Left hutch diverticulum with vesicoureteral reflux

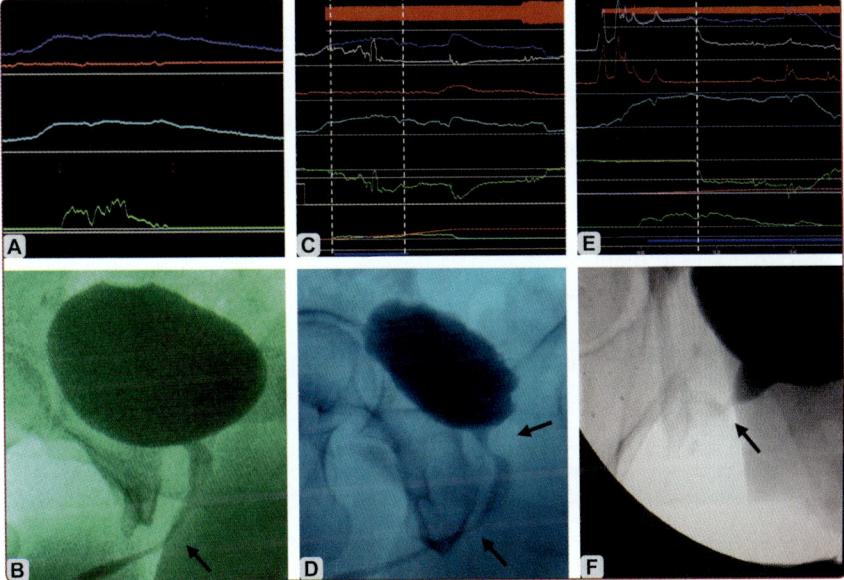

Figs 6A to F: Various instances of EUS dysfunction diagnosed on VCUG. (A-B) A 45-year-old male presented with voiding symptoms and constipation—UDS shows low pressure—low flow voiding with plateau detrusor pattern. VCUG confirms non-relaxation of EUS; (C-D) A 75-year-old male with L4–5 significant prolapse intervertebral disk presented with voiding symptoms—UDS shows moderate pressure—low flow voiding with irregular detrusor pattern. MUPP suggested double obstruction, both at bladder neck and EUS. VCUG confirmed double obstruction; (E-F) A 45-year-old female presented with urinary frequency and poor stream. UDS showed high pressure—low flow voiding with plateau detrusor pattern. MUPP suggested obstruction at midurethral level. VCUG confirmed non-relaxation of EUS with wide opening of bladder neck. Tracings—dark blue, Pves; white, Pura; red, Pabd; light blue, Pdet; green, Pclo; green, Q

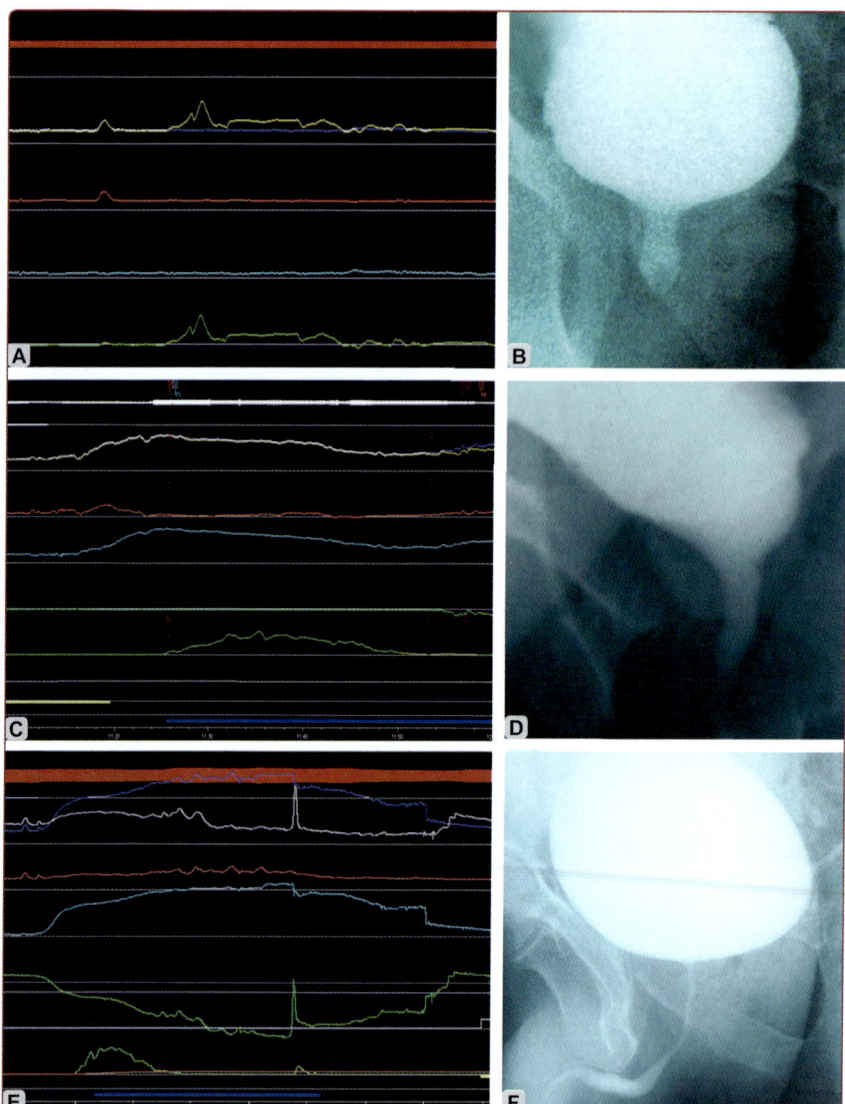

Figs 7A to F: Some clinical scenarios—(A-B) A 71-year-old male presented with obstructive nephropathy. Resting UPP showed very small low pressure profile (12mm, 45 cm H2O). Filling cystogram confirmed incompetent bladder neck. MUPP showed a high pressure – low flow voiding with plateau detrusor pattern and VCUG confirmed a non-relaxating EUS (not shown). (C-D) A 57-year-old female presented with obstructive nephropathy. UDS showed high pressure—low flow voiding. MUPP showed no evidence of BOO which was confirmed by VCUG; (E-F) A 65-year-old male presented with obstructive voiding symptoms with grade II enlarged prostate. UDS showed high pressure—low flow voiding with bell-shaped detrusor pattern. MUPP showed high grade prostatic obstruction. This was confirmed by VCUG. Tracings—dark blue, Pves; white, Pura; red, Pabd; light blue, Pdet; green, Pclo; green, Q

SUGGESTED READING

1. Twiss C, Fleschmann N, Nitti VW. Correlation of abdominal leak point pressure with objective incontinence severity in men with post radical prostatectomy stress incontinence. Neurourol Urodynam. 2005;24:207–10.

CHAPTER 6

Urethral Pressure Profilometry (UPP)

INTRODUCTION

UPP is indicated when the clinician is interested in knowing the function of the urethra. Similar to cystometry, urethral pressure can be measured using fluid infusion, air-charged or catheter-tip transducers. UPP is performed both during storage and voiding phase; during storage, it is performed during rest as well as stress maneuvers.

Over and above setup of cystometry, the additional requirements of UPP are—a special catheter, an automated electromechanical puller and an additional pressure transducer to record urethral pressure (Figures 1A to C). All types of catheters measure hydrostatic pressure, i.e. they require presence of water column at the pressure measurement port. For Pves, no specialized fluid irrigation is required, since it is placed in fluid-filled cavity both during filling and voiding phase. A competent urethra is not filled with fluid during filling phase. Therefore, an alternative arrangement must be made for irrigation of Pura channel; the resistance to this flow will be recorded as UPP.

Although urethral pressure can be measured using single or double lumen catheters, a triple-lumen catheter is most optimal for simultaneous measurement of bladder pressure (Pves) and urethral pressure (Pura), as

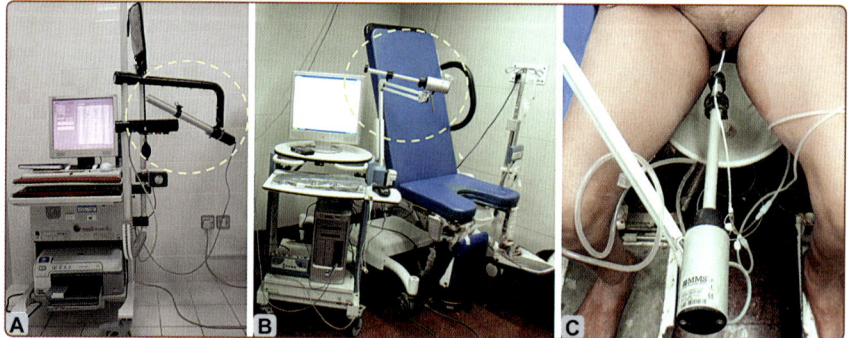

Figs 1A to C: Two urodynamic machines with dedicated motorized automated pullers (broken circle): (A) Mediwatch Duet at NMC specialty hospital, Abu Dhabi, UAE; (B) Solar Silver, MMS at PGIMER, Chandigarh, India; (C) A female patient undergoing UPP—the UPP catheter is clipped to the puller

well as fluid infusion. Two types of fluid infusion triple-lumen catheters are available (Figure 2):

a. In system 'a', Pves orifice is placed close to the tip and orifice of Infusion channel (inf) is placed just next to Pura ~5 cm distal to Pves. Both Inf and Pura orifices are surrounded by elevated ring plateaus on either side to facilitate infusion fluid to remain over Pura orifice for pressure reading. The same irrigation orifice is used for bladder filling.

b. In system 'b' orifice of infusion channel is at the tip (for filling bladder), followed by Pves channel (~1 cm distal) and Pura channel (~6 cm distal). For measuring Pura in empty urethra during filling phase, this channel is separately perfused continuously at ~0.5–1.0 mL/min using capillary tubing (Figures 3A and B).

The initial setup is same as that in cystometry, i.e. consent, sterile urine, prophylactic antibiotic, placement of rectal catheter, UPP catheter and EMG electrodes. The automated puller is placed facing the penis/introitus and the UPP catheter is attached to it. As per the above description depending on which type of UPP catheter has been used, the following circuit is connected:

The whole circuit is made air-free and zeroing is performed in standard fashion. UPP is most commonly performed in sitting position; however, depending on individual clinical requirements, positions can be changed and it can virtually be performed in any position (sitting, standing, squatting, supine).

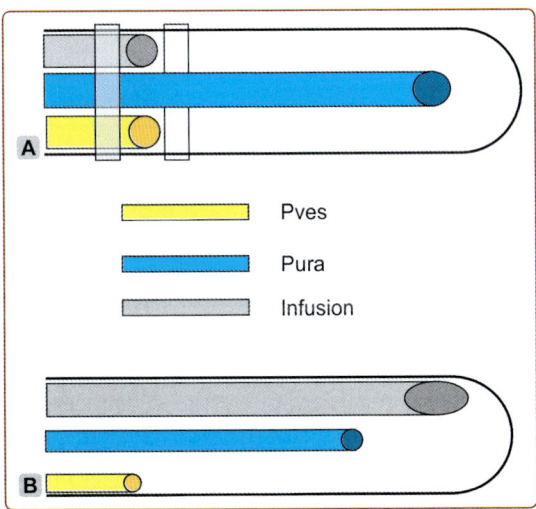

Fig. 2: In system 'a', Pves orifice is placed close to the tip and orifice of infusion channel is placed just next to Pura ~5 cm distal to Pves. Both Inf and Pura orifices are surrounded by elevated ring-plateaus on either side to facilitate infusion fluid to remain over Pura orifice for pressure reading. The same irrigation orifice is used for bladder filling. In system 'b', orifice of infusion channel is at the tip (for filling bladder), followed by Pves channel (~1 cm distal) and Pura channel (~6 cm distal). For measuring Pura in empty urethra during filling phase, this channel is separately perfused continuously at ~0.5–1.0 mL/min using capillary tubing

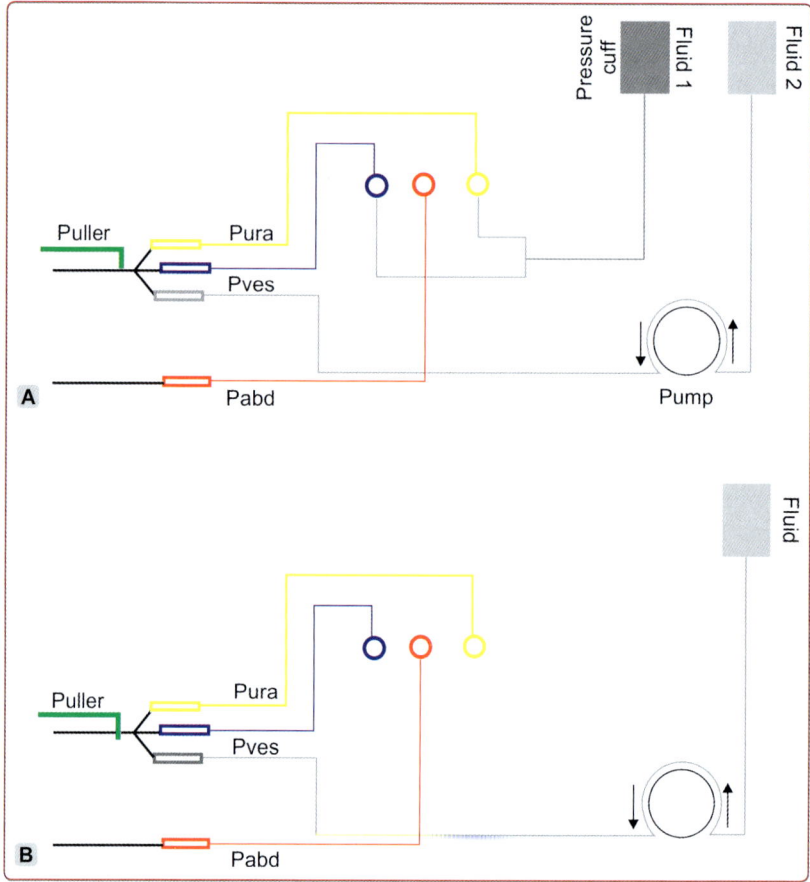

Figs 3A and B: Connection circuits for UPP using 3-lumen catheters. (A) Setup using catheter b (with tip infusion type design); and (B) Setup using catheter a (with tip Pves measurement type design)

Bladder filling is initiated through infusion channel (light grey) at physiological fill rate (discussed in cystometry chapter). After filling ~50–150 mL, depending presence or absence of detrusor overactivity and poor compliance, resting urethral pressure profile is recorded. In circuit (a) (with pressure cuff) pump infusion is stopped and pressure cuff infusion (at 300 mm Hg pressure) is started via capillary extension lines into Pura and Pves channels; this provides infusion rate ~0.5–1.0 mL/min (Figure 3a). At this time, puller is started to pull at a modifiable predefined rate (typically 2 mm/s; desired rate 1–4 mm/s). In circuit (b), the pump infusion is slowed down to 2–6 mL/s; no additional pressure pumping is required (Figure 3b). The advantage of circuit (b) is that it is simple to use. The advantage of circuit (a) is that bladder infusion can continue with simultaneous recording of Pura.

As soon as the orifice of Pura channel enters bladder neck, the infusion is met with resistance of urethral wall reflecting as a positive deflection on the computer screen. It's value indicates static pressure at that particular point. With continued pulling, the whole urethral pressure profile (posterior urethra in men and entire urethra in women) is recorded. Profile end is marked when Pura tracing crosses Pves tracing (i.e. Pclo becomes zero). Typical resting profile of a man and woman is described in Figures 4A and B. If puller is not available, catheter can be pulled manually each time by 5–10 mm and each pull is marked on the screen. Although not as accurate as automated puller, meaningful derivations can be made.

> **Tip**
>
> If the length of posterior urethra is more than the distance between Pura and Pves orifice (i.e. ~5 cm), one should continue to pull till whole posterior urethra has been negotiated and interpretation should be based on Pura tracing (and not Pclo); some approximations have to be made. Similar situation arises when patient develops detrusor overactivity during recording of the resting profile (Figures 5A and B).

Two important parameters are described in RUPP:
a. *Urethral profile length*—As in Figures 4A and B, male-profile can be divided into prostatic and sphincter zone. The following deviations need special mention:
   1. In patients with prostatic enlargement, the prostatic profile tends to be longer and has higher pressure.

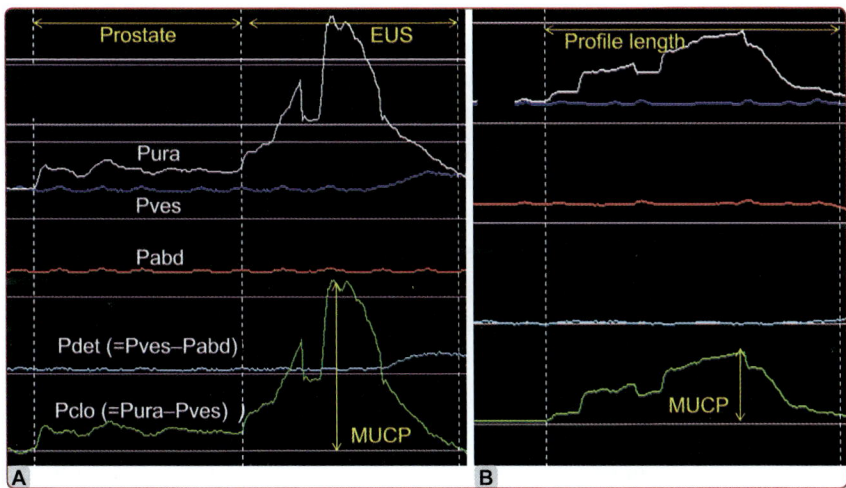

Figs 4A and B: Resting urethral pressure profile: (A) Male—plateau of prostatic zone, with steep rise of pressure in external urethral sphincter region (EUS). The prostatic pressure tends to be higher in men with BPH; (B) Female—asymmetrical bell shaped curve with no clear zonal demarcation. Tracings—dark blue, Pves; white, Pura; red, Pabd; light blue, Pdet; green, Pclo

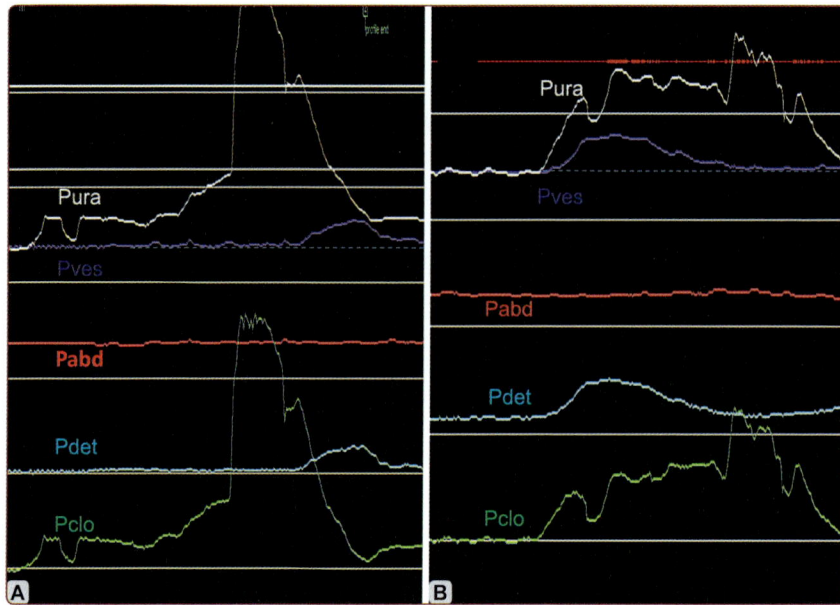

Figs 5A and B: Artifact caused by changes in Pves recording. (A) A long-resting UPP of a 34-year-old man with dysfunctional elimination syndrome—a rise in Pves toward the end of the profile is due to Pves orifice coming into urethra; (B) a resting UPP of a 36-year-old male with overactive bladder—a rise in Pves due to DO during recording of profile. In both the situations, Pura and not Pclo tracing should be used for interpretation. It would be helpful to draw an imaginary baseline on Pves (dashed line). Tracings—dark blue, Pves; white, Pura; red, Pabd; light blue, Pdet; green, Pclo

2. In patients with extrinsic sphincter deficiency after radical cystoprostatectomy or prostatectomy, a continuous low pressure plateau is observed which does not fall to baseline. Possible explanation is increased tone and activity (compensatory) of bulbospongiosus muscle to compensate for sphincter deficiency. To note, in normal individuals, the muscle responsible for voluntary interruption of stream is bulbospongiosus (followed by pelvic floor).
3. Patients with established lower motor neuron type of neurogenic bladder (e.g. meningomyelocele) tend to have a small low amplitude bell-shaped profile, which is suggestive of incompetent bladder neck (which does not show) and fixed EUS tone.

b. *Maximum urethral closure pressure (MUCP):* Urethral closure pressure is urethral pressure over and above bladder pressure (Pclo = Pura − Pves). Similar to Pdet, this is not measured directly but derived from the above equation by the software on real-time basis. The maximum value of Pclo (= MUCP) is a clinically useful parameter associated with status of continence. Generally, it is located at the level of EUS in both sexes. Normal values of MUCP widely vary between individuals. In men, mean values

are in the range of 70s cm H2O (vary from 30s to 120s) and change a little with age. Whereas, in women, the mean values tend to drop by 8–10 cm H2O with each quarter of life from mean of 90 (age <25 years) to 65 (age >64 years). Two deviations need to be mentioned:
1. Very low MUCP—In women with stress urinary incontinence, MUCP <20–30 cm H2O is considered to be indicative of instrinsic sphincter deficiency which may have implication in type of treatment offered (suspension versus sling); however, a large overlap is present.
2. Very high MUCP—In patients with pelvic floor dysfunction and dysfunctional elimination syndrome, MUCP tends to be very high, commonly >150 cm H2O. Notably, such high MUCP can be observed even in anxious patients who are voluntarily contracting pelvic floor. To overcome this artifact, the patient is encouraged to relax and the resting profile is repeated to insure reproducibility; in case of different readings, the one with lower MUCP is chosen (most relaxed profile).

c. *Urethral relaxation incontinence:* This is measured during resting UPP cycle. Previously known as urethral instability, it is an uncommon phenomenon, sometimes detected in women presenting with large volume urinary leakage without prior warning/urgency. It is defined as a fall of Pura >15 cm H2O during filling without concomitant rise in abdominal pressure or detrusor overactivity. Alternatively, maximum urethral pressure variation ratio of 33% or more (ΔMUPX100/highest MUP) is considered indicative of this condition. It is not clear whether or not, it is a variant of a prematurely activated micturition reflex, in which the rise in detrusor pressure due to an involuntary contraction is too small to see. According to the ICS, it is better to give a full description, if symptoms are seen in association with a decrease in urethral pressure during cystometry.

STRESS UPP

Stress UPP is required in patients who have LUT dysfunction in abdominal stress phase, i.e. with stress urinary incontinence. Once the resting profile is recorded, the catheter is adjusted with puller or manually, so that Pura orifice is placed just distal to the MUCP point (corresponding to distal part of EUS). To note, Pves orifice and infusion orifice are in the bladder only. Filling is continued till the bladder volume ~200 mL and stress profile is recorded in a similar fashion as described in leak point pressure section of cystometry. The interpretation is as under:

Leak Point Pressure

Investigators have tried to overcome the limitation of measuring ALPP with cystometry by using stress UPP. If the perfusion is off, Pura recording shows a low pressure. If the patient leaks on cough or valsalva, urine will come in the urethra and a water column with bladder pressure will form in the urethra. This sudden rise in Pura is recorded on the tracing. The Pves at the transition point is CLPP/VLPP. This is particularly important in CLPP; during cystometry, only the peak Pves of cough which led to leak can be taken as CLPP, whereas, the patient might have started leaking anywhere during the crescendo phase. This limitation is overcome in UPP where the transition point of Pura can exactly mark the point on crescendo of Pves (CLPP) (Figures 6A and B).

Unfortunately, despite being promising, this method has not been studied extensively and its CLPP/VLPP reference values are not standardized.

Pressure Transmission Ratio

Urethral axial hypermobility (UH) is an important clinical finding in patients with SUI. It is diagnosed by Q-tip test; with patient in lithotomy position, a Q-tip (e.g. sterilized ear bud) is inserted into urethra and patient is asked to strain.

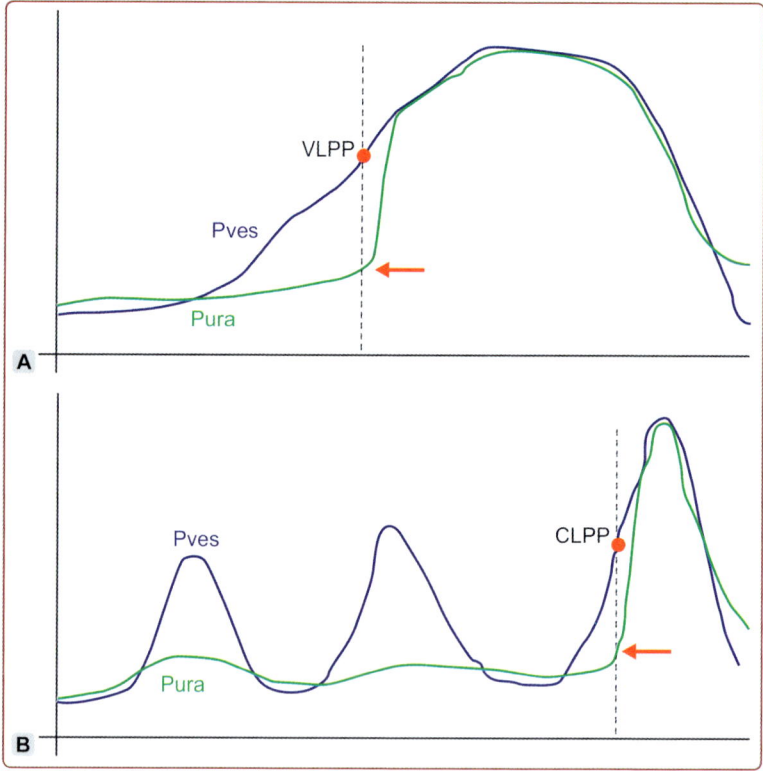

Figs 6A and B: UPP method of measuring abdominal leak point pressures. It potentially overcomes the delay in perceiving the leak (either direct visually or fluoroscopically). The point on Pves tracing (red-dot) corresponding to sudden pressure rise in Pura tracing (red arrow) corresponds to VLPP (A) or CLPP (B).

UH is said to be present when this Q-tip rotates upto an angle >30–35 degrees from horizontal. In a patient with SUI, its presence indicates genuine stress incontinence because of the weakness of pelvic floor support.

Investigators have made attempts to make objective assessment of presence, and grade the UH by UPP. With UPP catheter in situ (same status as described), the infusion is turned on in Pura as in resting profile. The patient is asked to strain/cough and change in Pves and Pura is noted. The patient should not leak during this recording; else intraluminal Pves recording will occur representing ALPP. Pressure transmission ratio (PTR) is defined by the following equation:

$$PTR = \Delta Pura \times 100/\Delta Pves$$

This calculation is available in various UDS softwares as an automatic function, or it can be performed manually. In real-time, UH is seen as a negative deflection in Pclo (= Pura – Pves) tracing (Figures 7A and B)

It is believed that in presence of UH, mid-urethra tends to prolapse out of pelvic floor support and therefore, transmission of pressure to this part of urethra is less than the abdominal pressure. It is estimated that a PTR <70% is indicative of UH. Unfortunately, PTR has remained as an orphan concept and has not been widely studied.

MICTURITIONAL UPP (MUPP)

The diagnosis and localization of urinary outflow obstruction is fundamental to the practice of urology. Apart from in symptomatic men in BPH age group

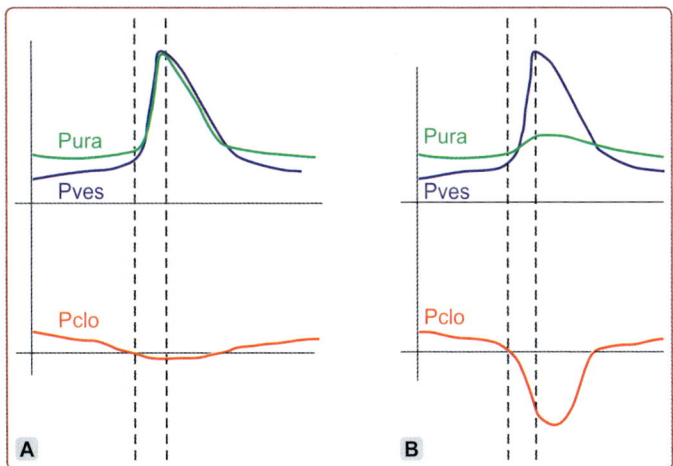

Figs 7A and B: Pressure-transmission ratio. (A) Normal–complete pressure transmission evident by similar rise in Pura and Pves during cough; Pclo (=Pura-Pves) is zero; (B) Abnormal—poor pressure transmission evident by small rise in Pura with cough; Pclo shows a negative deflection

without significant neurological disorders (diabetes mellitus, parkinsonism, cerebrovascular accident, etc.) and most patients with urethral stricture disease, practically, in every other patient presenting with voiding dysfunction, it is important to diagnose and localize functional bladder outlet obstruction (BOO) for appropriate management, particularly, when invasive treatment is being planned (e.g. bladder neck incision, TURP, sphincterotomy, botox®, neuromodulation).

In the last chapter, we have seen that various parameters of urethral resistance relations have been studied for diagnosis of BOO. Many of these parameters are complex in understanding, computation, and interpretation and have not been validated for common usage; lastly, apart from CHESS graph, none of these point toward etiology of the problem. In case of doubtful results, video UDS has been employed to diagnose and localize BOO; a diagnosis by visualization of anatomy.

The concept of MUPP is based on Bernaulli's principle, which states that as a fluid passes through a pipe that narrows or widens, the velocity and pressure of the fluid vary. As the pipe narrows, the fluid flows more quickly and it is accompanied by fall in static pressure. Therefore, if we can measure the pressure in bladder and urethra during the act of voiding, we can diagnose and localize the BOO. Plausibly, this is a direct and straightforward functional method for this purpose, inasmuch as video UDS.

To perform MUPP, once the resting profile has been recorded, the UPP catheter is pulled back to the bladder neck (marked by elevation of Pura over Pves) and stopped there. The filling cystometry is continued as described in previous chapter. Once micturition command is given and urine flow starts, the puller is turned on, so that it negotiates the urethra, recording the Pura all along in real-time. We typically keep the puller speed to 2 mm/sec.

> **Tip**
>
> During voiding, puller is stopped once the Pura orifice is estimated to have negotiated past the EUS; it is an approximation based on the resting profile length (Figure 8). Stopping is important, since continued pulling may bring the Pves orifice into bladder neck confounding the results of Pclo (i.e. Pura – Pves).

Normal voiding profile results are as follows (Figures 9A and B):
a. *Males:* There is no/minimal (<5 cm H2O) pressure gradient along the prostatic urethra (i.e. Pclo 0). A drop of Pura upto 20 cm H2O at the level of EUS is acceptable in patients with otherwise normal voiding pattern. This artifact happens due to obstruction of least dilatable part of urethra (i.e. membranous) caused by the catheter *per se*.

Chapter 6 Urethral Pressure Profilometry (UPP)

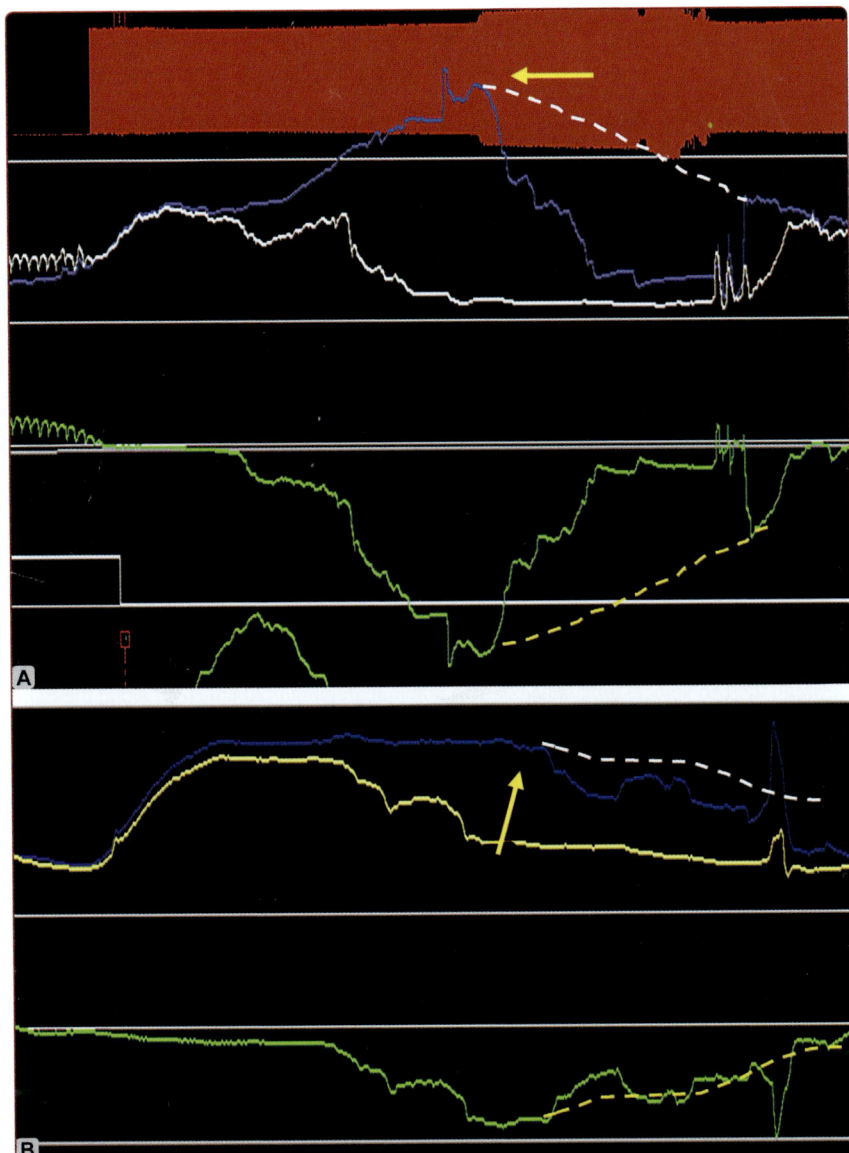

Fig. 8: Artifacts arising during MUPP out of Pves orifice coming into posterior urethra in patients with prostatic obstruction. Solid arrows mark the point at which Pves orifice entered into obstructed prostatic urethra and showed an irregularly shaped fall in Pves. Broken white lines represent the approximate true Pves line had it remained in bladder; broken yellow lines represent approximate true tracing of Pclo after correction

b. *Females:* There is no/minimal (<5 cm H2O) pressure gradient in any part of urethra (i.e. Pclo 0). A minor dip in Pura at the level of urethral meatus may be observed.

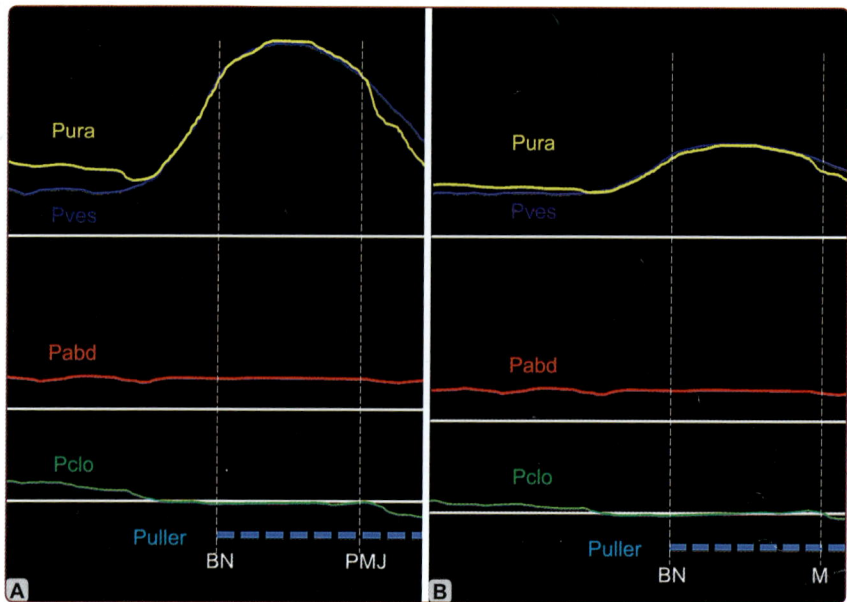

Figs 9A and B: Linear diagrammatic representation of normal micturitional urethral pressure profile in (A) Male—no Pura—Pves (= Pclo) pressure gradient along the prostatic urethra, i.e. between the two vertical broken lines and a nominal gradient (<20 cm H2O) along the EUS; (B) Female—no Pura – Pves (= Pclo) pressure gradient along the entire urethra till close to meatus where minimal drop is observed (undefined). BN = bladder neck, PMJ = prostate-membranous junction, M = meatus

Any pressure gradient >5 cm H2O (Pclomax < –5 cm H2O) along prostatic urethra in male and along entire urethra in female (except for terminal few millimetre) is diagnostic of BOO. The numerical value of gradient (Pclo) is indicative of degree of BOO, and the point at which gradient appears marks the most proximal level of obstruction (Figures 10A and C).

Definition is less clear for obstruction at the level of EUS in males. Generally, a gradient >20–30 cm H2O (Pclo< –20–30) is considered indicative of obstruction at that level. However, there is a caveat in this simplex. Often, patients with pelvic floor dysfunction (EUS dysfunction) demonstrate low pressure-low flow type of void with plateau detrusor pattern; therefore, the pressure head, i.e. Pves itself is low. In this situation, even a drop of 20 cm H2O or less will indicate obstruction, since the percentage fall of Pura below Pves may be quite high (Figures 10B and D).

In females, diagnosis and localization of BOO has been more straightforward irrespective of location. In fact, we have been able to exclude the diagnosis of BOO in some women, even when pressure-flow parameters indicated otherwise. Some representative patterns are represented in Figures 11A to F.

Chapter 6 Urethral Pressure Profilometry (UPP)

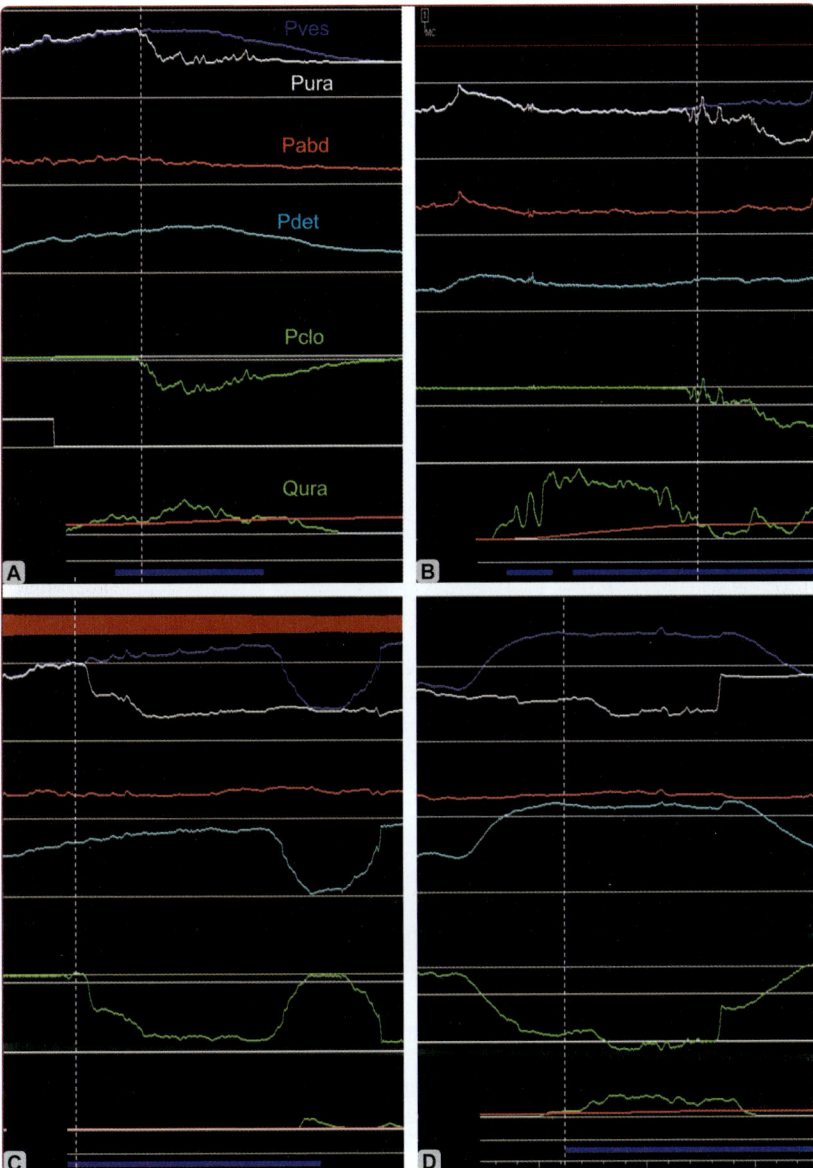

Figs 10A to D: Some abnormal patterns of micturitional UPP in men. Vertical broken white lines represent proximal level of obstruction. The obstruction is seen as a downward deflection in Pura compared to Pves and deflection of Pclo tracing below baseline. All the diagnoses were confirmed with voiding cystourethrogram. (A) A 65-year-old male with clinical prostatic enlargement with severe obstructive symptoms. High pressure—low flow voiding pattern and obstruction starting few millimetre from bladder neck; (B) A 27-year-old male with dysfunctional elimination syndrome. Low pressure-low flow voiding with plateau pattern of Pdet and obstruction at EUS. To note, numerical value of Pura-Pves gradient is just under 20 cm H2O; however, in presence of a low pressure head of Pves, Pura is seen to fall nearly to baseline, thus, suggesting obstruction at that level; (C) A 38-year-old male with primary bladder neck obstruction, showing obstruction starting right from bladder neck. A sudden dip in Pves in the later part of the tracing indicates position of Pves orifice of the triple-lumen catheter into prostatic urethra thus, displaying urethral pressure. To note, restoration of the Pves toward the end is the result of reposition of the catheter, so that Pves orifice is placed back in bladder; (D) A 42-year-old male with voiding dysfunction and constipation. He demonstrated high pressure-low flow voiding with plateau detrusor pattern. The obstruction started right from the bladder neck but also had non-relaxation of EUS, a case of double obstruction (BN>EUS)

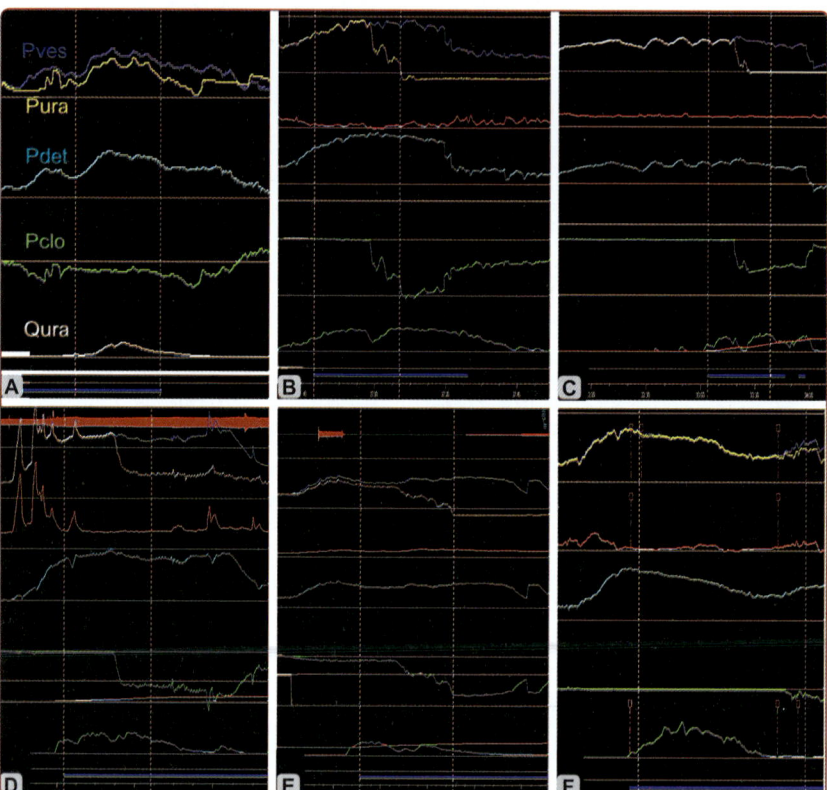

Figs 11A to F: Some abnormal patterns of Micturitional UPP in women. Broken vertical lines represent profile length marked according to the results of resting profile. The obstruction is seen as a downward deflection in Pura compared to Pves and deflection of Pclo tracing below baseline. All the diagnosis were confirmed with voiding cystourethrogram. (A) A 68-year-old female with bladder neck obstruction. Calibration easy with 18F foley catheter. Moderately high pressure-low flow voiding; Pclo is below baseline right from bladder neck and maintained throughout the profile. (B) A 73-year-old female with distal urethral narrowing; 18Fr foley catheter admitting snugly. High pressure-low flow voiding with obstruction starting past middle of urethra. (C) A 30-year-old female with dysfunctional elimination syndrome. Calibration easy with 18F foley catheter. Low pressure-low flow voiding with plateau detrusor pattern. Obstruction starting approximately in the mid-urethra corresponding to EUS. (D) A 46-year-old female with marked frequency and poor voiding. Calibration easy with 18F foley catheter. High pressure-low flow voiding with plateau detrusor pattern. Obstruction starting at mid-urethra corresponding to EUS. (E) A 58-year-old female with voiding dysfunction. Calibration snug with 18F foley catheter. Moderate pressure-low flow voiding with obstruction starting at bladder neck (low grade) becoming marked at mid-urethra; a case of double obstruction. (F) A 62-year-old female with urgency, poor stream and obstructive uropathy. High pressure-low flow voiding pattern with no evidence of obstruction in urethra. Distal urethra showing a physiological fall of Pura by few cm H2O. She was successfully managed with anticholinergics

CHAPTER 7

Ambulatory UDS

As the name suggests, ambulatory UDS (AUDS) is a urodynamic study performed while the patient is ambulant. AUDS is required when questions remain unanswered even after office UDS and further treatment can change with further investigation. This is particularly true in defining the cause of incontinence in women.

Even if conducted at low flow rates, most of the time, filling rate during office UDS is much higher than natural rate of urine production (approximately 1mL/min or less). Such rapid filling rates may alter bladder behavior. For example—DO can be induced by rapid filling, cold filling solution and foreign body (catheter); patient may not be able to pass urine in unfamiliar surroundings of UDS lab and 'too-fast' muscle reorganization with rapid stretch of detrusor may lead to impaired detrusor contractility. Nevertheless, clinically meaningful results are obtained with office UDS in most circumstances.

Common situations where diagnosis remains in doubt after office UDS, AUDS may be helpful as follows:

a. Patient with incontinence, not demonstrable during office UDS.
b. Patient with urge incontinence, without demonstrable DO during office UDS (to differentiate between urethral-relaxation from DO).
c. Patient with voiding dysfunction, not able to void during office UDS.

The equipment of AUDS has been reasonably miniaturized in the past decades and with the advent of air-charged catheters, the recording has become easier (Figure 1). Many manufacturers provide the facility of AUDS software compatible with their office UDS machines. The following hardware and software are required to conduct the AUDS:

1. A portable pressure recorder with the following facilities:
   a. Record 2 or 3 pressures (Pves, Pabd, Pura)
   b. Preferably perineal integrated surface EMG
   c. Event marking buttons
   d. Leakage marker using urethral conductance
   e. Connectability to uroflowmeter.
2. A desktop/laptop computer.
3. Software to download and analyze the recorded data on a computer.

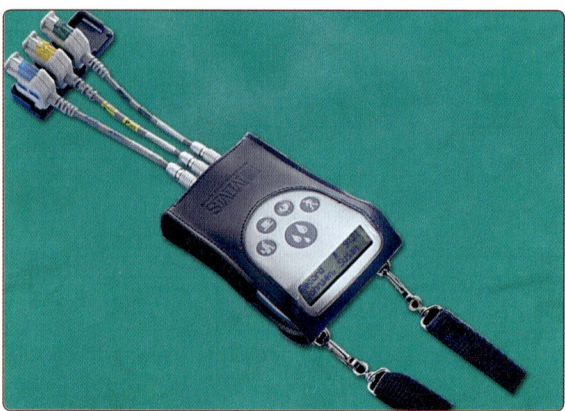

Fig. 1: Ambulatory urodynamic system (Luna®, MMS International, Enschede, the Netherlands). The recorder and T-DOC transducers. *(reproduced with permission from Technomed Medical Systems, sole distributors of MMS International, the Netherlands)*

4. Facility to connect by wireless technology (e.g. Bluetooth) is preferable.
5. A uroflowmeter.
6. Air-charged (T-DOC) catheters with transducers.

TECHNIQUE

Patient must be educated about the need for the test and be re-emphasized the importance of keeping catheters in place and 'marking' events in real-time. Once the catheters and electrodes are secured in place, the recorder is connected and worn on body in a pouch. The instrument is calibrated and all pressures are zeroed before activating the study. Typically, recording is done for about three hours. The patient is asked to move around in the hospital and do some activity cycles. The following cycles are recommended (Figures 2A to D):

a. *Resting*—when patient sits on chair (or lies down).
b. *Ambulant*—when patient moves about in the hospital.
c. *Stress*—when patient performs maneuvers which increase intra-abdominal pressure (e.g. coughing, straining, lifting weight, walking stairs, or any activity which brings about leakage in their routine).

   Detection of leakage can be done by one of the many ways—patient's perception, electric nappy, temperature sensitive nappy, urethral pressure measurement, urethral electrical conductance; none of these methods is foolproof.

d. *Voiding*—it is always preferable to conduct this part to complete urodynamic information, so that maximum information can be gathered

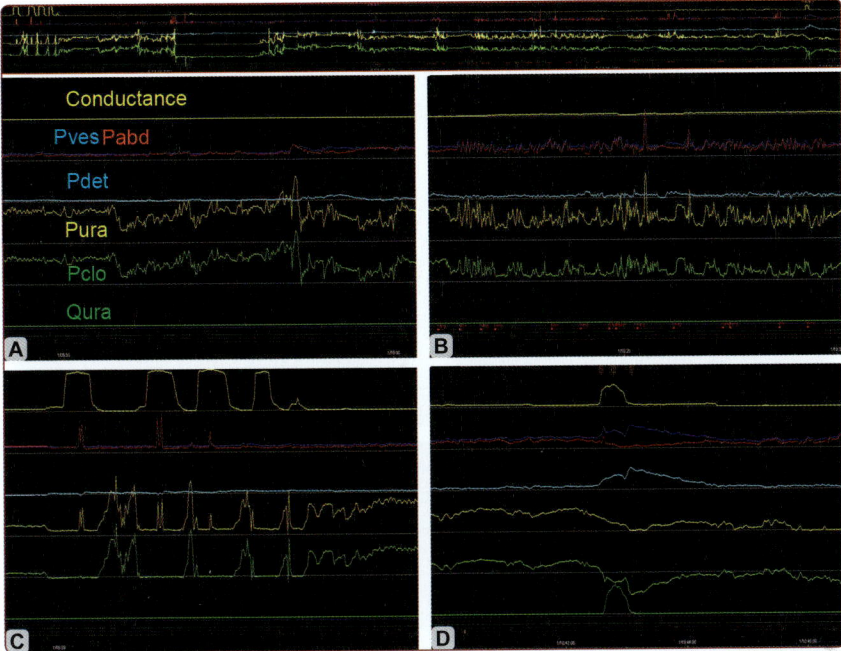

Figs 2A to D: A one hour tracing (top strip) of ambulatory urodynamic study demonstrating all the cycles (A) Resting phase—identifiable by quiescent Pves and Pabd tracings. Pura is turbulent representing variable urethral pressures; (B) Ambulant—identifiable by spiky Pves and Pabd. Low amplitude DO is appreciable on Pdet; (C) Stress—identifiable by spikes in Pves, Pabd as well as Pura (by virtue of a fluid bridge formed at that time). To note, the deflection in top tracing (conductance) reflects presence of fluid between two urethral ring electrodes; (D) Voiding—AUDS was connected to uroflowmeter. Low pressure-high flow voiding reflecting normal voiding phase

from this painstaking investigation. Patient is asked to report whenever they wish to urinate. The AUDS is connected to the desktop (or directly to the uroflowmeter), so that a synchronized recording of pressure flow is taken.

INTERPRETATION

Interpretation of AUDS can be challenging and requires expertize and experience (Figures 3A and B). Calibration may not be maintained well, catheter might move from correct position, particularly the Pura channel, patient may not have inserted marker at the correct time and voiding may have taken place without a synchronized uroflowmeter.

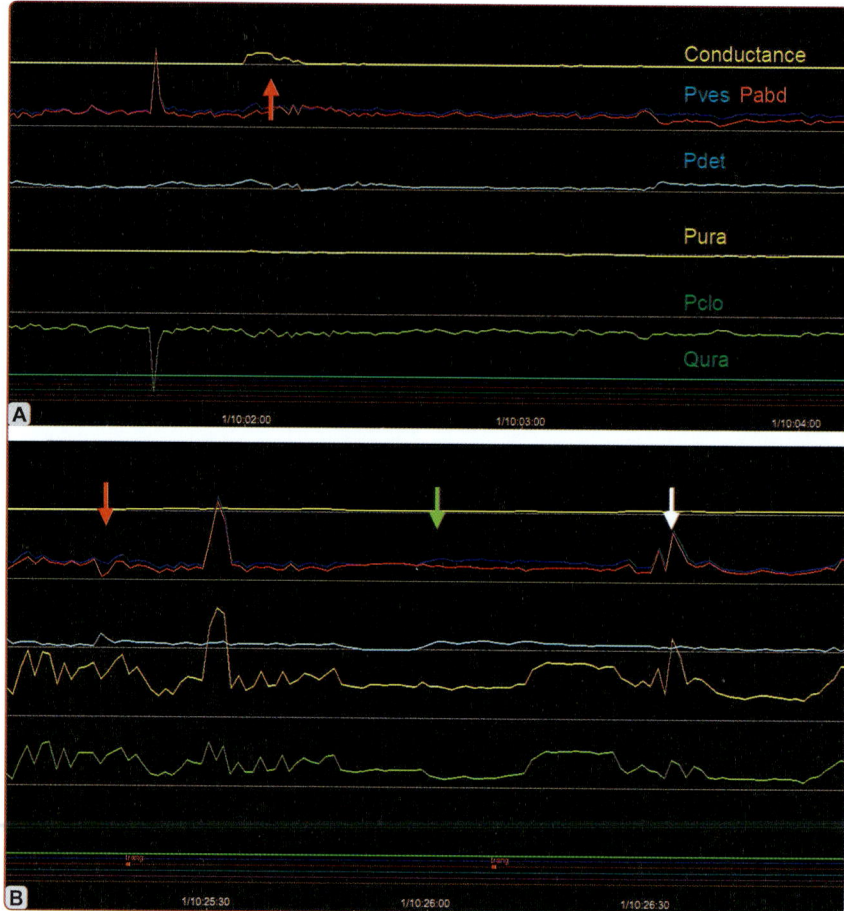

Figs 3A and B: Interpretation of AUDS requires a patient review of the whole tracing in zoom mode to identify artifacts and avoid incorrect interpretation. (A) An artifactual recording in conductance electrode. A baseline recording of Pura is notable (compare with graph B in which it shows a variable positive value). No event was marked at this point; (B) Red arrow—artifactual recording of DO (Pdet), which is due to negative deflection of Pabd. Green arrow—a true recording of DO (Pdet), which is due to positive deflection in Pves. White arrow—a well-maintained zeroing

CHAPTER 8

Whitaker Test

INTRODUCTION

Whitaker test also known as antegrade pressure measurement (APM) or perfusion flow study. It is a method of antegrade measurement of pressure in the upper urinary tract. It was first described by Whitaker in 1973 and was designed to establish whether or not urinary tract dilatation is caused by obstruction [1]. The test can be used to investigate a suspected ureteropelvic junction (UPJ) obstruction or ureterovesical junction (UVJ) obstruction. Isotope scan and ultrasound sometimes fail to give a definitive answer whether the hydronephrosis represents a dilated or an obstructed system. This may be the case in kidneys with a severe impairment of function, in patients with bilateral dilated upper tracts and in patients with lower ureteral obstruction. In kidneys with a huge dilatation or with a differential function of less than 20%, both renogram and MRI can fail to give a definitive diagnosis. In these cases, Whitaker test can discriminate between non-obstructive and obstructive dilatation.

A sterile urine culture should be insured before the test, since there is real risk of bacteremia during the test. We give prophylactic antibiotic covering common gram negative organisms just before the test. A bowel preparation according to local practice should be done if the test is to be performed under fluoroscopic guidance with iodinated contrast material.

PROCEDURE

During Whitaker test, the differential pressure across a suspected obstruction is measured (Figure 1). Firstly, a 6Fr single lumen catheter (e.g. infant feeding tube) is placed inside the bladder, and a 6Fr double lumen cystometry catheter is placed into the renal pelvis through a previously established nephrostomy tract; alternatively, if facility is available, a 3Fr microtip catheter is placed through a percutaneous needle into the renal pelvis. Similar to cystometry, the catheter is connected to transducer ($P_{pelvis} \equiv P_{ves}$ channel) and infusion pump of the urodynamic system. The catheter in the bladder is also connected to the pressure transducer ($P_{bladder} \equiv P_{abd}$ channel). The patient is placed in supine position and zeroing is performed at pubic symphysis level. To note, it does not matter in interpretation as to which level we are zeroing, since the interpretable variable (intrapelvic pressure IPP = Pves − Pabd) is a difference between two variables zeroed at the same level similar to Pdet.

Once the apparatus is setup (Figure 1), infusion of normal saline (or 30% meglumine-diatrizoate solution if fluoroscopy is to be performed) is started from renal pelvic catheter at a rate of 10 mL/min saline. The Ppelvis and Pbladder are measured in real-time and IPP calculated in real-time, much like Pdet (Figure 2). During the study, the filling state of both the renal pelvis and the bladder is controlled by ultrasound or fluoroscopy to make sure that a steady state of dilatation has been reached; bladder over-distension is to be avoided at any cost.

INTERPRETATION OF RESULTS

At the filling rate of 10 mL/min, the following interpretations can be made—
  i. Differential pressures (IPP) <15 cm H2O: unobstructed
  ii. IPP 15–22 cm H2O: indeterminate
  iii. IPP > 22 cm H2O: obstructed

Obviously, in category I and III results, the interpretation is straightforward and management can be definitively directed. In the category II, the management is more dubious and directed by clinical suspicion.

ROLE OF WHITAKER TEST

1. Equivocal results from less invasive tests.
2. Suspected obstruction with poor kidney function.

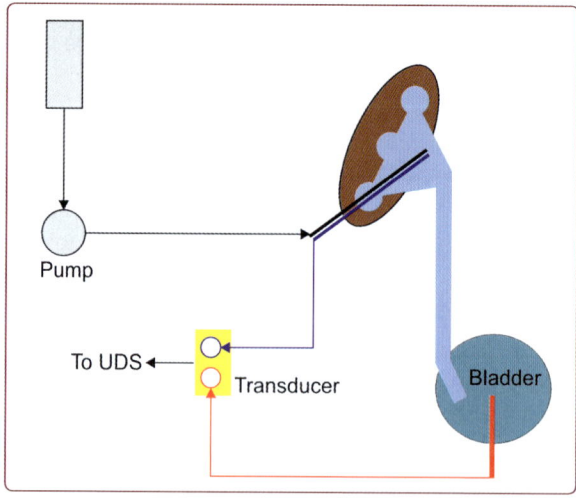

Fig. 1: Simplified circuit of upper tract urodynamic study

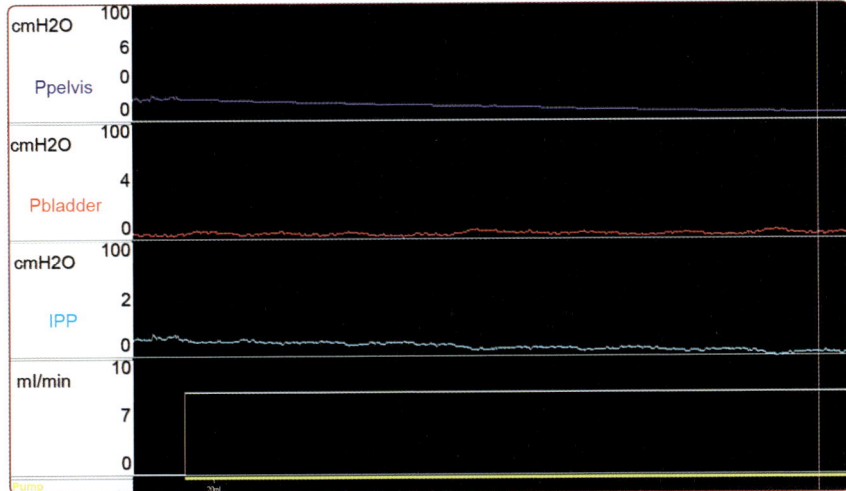

Fig. 2: Graphical representation of upper tract UDS. Ppelvis—pressure in renal pelvis; Pbladder—bladder pressure, IPP—true intrapelvic pressure (= Ppelvis − Pbladder)

3. Loin pain with a negative diuresis renogram (in the event of poor renal function, the diuretic renogram may be falsely negative, because the diuretic may not sufficiently raise the urine flow).
4. Suspected intermittent obstruction.
5. Gross dilatation with a positive diuresis renogram.

DRAWBACKS OF WHITAKER TEST

1. It does not actually define or measure obstruction. It only records the pressure in the renal pelvis during non-physiologically high flow rates. Under most circumstances, such high rates of urine production may never be encountered. Therefore, even if a system is deemed obstructed by Whitaker test at a rate of 10 mL/min, it may be falsely positive in clinical perspective. Therefore, in case we get an obstructed result, we repeat the test at lower filling rate (e.g. 6–7 mL/m) and try to interpret the changes in IPP clinically.
2. There is also a risk that the test is terminated before the pelvicalyceal system is full, that is before a steady state is reached. Hence, ultrasound control or fluoroscopy is needed during pressure measurement to make sure that a true steady state has been reached.
3. Invasive nature of the test. During placement of the needle in the pelvicalyceal system, chance of vascular injury leading to bleeding and hematoma formation, injury to colon or pleural cavity might occur.
4. Radiation exposure.

SUGGESTED READING

1. Djurhuus JC, Sorensen SS, Jorgensen TM, et al. Predictive value of pressure flow studies for the functional outcome of reconstructive surgery for hydronephrosis. Br J Urol. 1985;57:6–9.
2. Whitaker RH, Buxton-Thomas MS. A comparison of pressure flow studies and renography in equivocal upper urinary tract obstruction. J Urol. 1984;131:446.
3. Whitaker RH. Methods of assessing obstruction in dilated ureters. Br J Urol. 1973;45:15–22.

CHAPTER 9

Representative Case Discussion

PATIENT 1

A 32-year-old male presented with severe obstructive LUTS, along with severe left-side backache while voiding. His bladder diary was unremarkable.

Examination

Abdominal—NAD
Genital—NAD
FNE—NAD
DRE—NAD

Uroflowmetry

Showed obstructive type low flow pattern (Qmax 6 mL/s, Qave 4 mL/s, VV 161 mL, PVR 0 mL) [Figure 1A]

Considering his severe symptoms, he qualified for a UDS and underwent MUPP (for presence, degree and location of BOO) as well as VCUG (for verification of finding on MUPP and to look for anatomical defect in LUT).

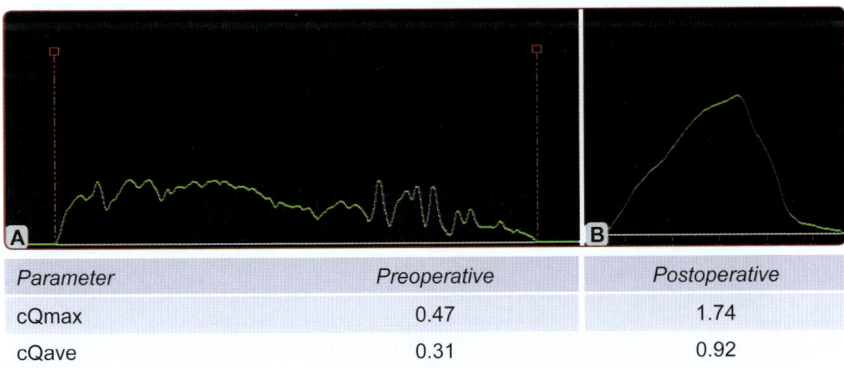

Parameter	Preoperative	Postoperative
cQmax	0.47	1.74
cQave	0.31	0.92

Figs 1A and B: Uroflowmetry of patient 1 (A) at presentation; (B) after endoscopic treatment

Pressure-flow Analysis

High-pressure, low-flow voiding pattern. PdetQmax – 128 cm H2O, Pdetmax – 177 cm H2O, Qmax – 6 mL/s, Qave – 4 mL/s, PVR – 0 mL. Plateau pattern of detrusor contraction: point toward EUS dysfunction.

AG number – 116, DAMPF – 99, OCO – 2.46, curvature 0.83, CHESS location – D3 (indicative of bladder neck obstruction).

UPP (Figure 2A)

Description of Resting Profile

Profile length—41 mm total, 28 mm prostatic, 13 mm EUS. MUCP – 143 cm H2O (in EUS zone).

Description of Micturitional Profile

Pclo(Prostatic urethra) : –10 to –14 cm H2O
Pclo(EUS) : –152 cm H2O. Patient had severe pain in left flank during voiding and, therefore, he tried to stop urination.

VCUG done on the same day reproduced the MUPP findings—bladder neck and EUS obstruction. It also showed left hutch diverticulum with reflux explaining pain during voiding (Figure 2B).

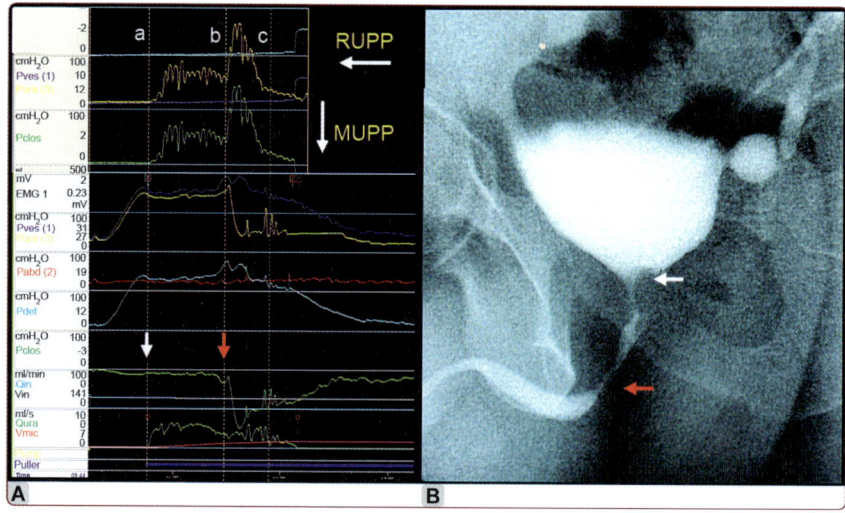

Figs 2A and B: Urodynamics of patient 1 (A) urethral pressure profilometry—point a represents bladder neck and b-c, EUS; (B) MCU reveals double obstruction, white arrow represents obstruction at bladder neck and red arrow obstruction at EUS

Interpretation

Neurologically, intact young man with voiding dysfunction and left flank pain during voiding. Unquestionably, there is bladder overactivity and presence of severe bladder outlet obstruction. Detrusor pattern, MUPP and VCUG indicate presence of dual obstruction, i.e. both at the bladder neck and the EUS. The question is which one to treat first, the bladder neck or the EUS.

Since the patient has no neurological affliction, has no defecation dysfunction, has definitive BN obstruction, very high pressure and low flow voiding, voluntary EUS squeezing by the patient to abort voiding in view of pain, the EUS dysfunction seen in this study is most likely secondary (voluntary). This is further supported by high foot-point and steep pressure-flow graph on CHESS plot, which indicates bladder neck obstruction.

This patient underwent cystoscopy and transurethral incision of prostate. He responded favorably in terms of improvement in flow (Figure 1B) and abolition of pain. He does have urgency for which medical management has been instituted.

PATIENT 2

A 36-year-old male presented with voiding symptoms ever since he remembers. He had undergone fulguration of posterior urethral valves in 2006, following which he had improved. In 2007, the symptoms recurred following bilateral ureteral reimplantation done for persistent reflux. He first presented to our institution in 2011 with symptoms of sensation of incomplete evacuation and poor stream.

Examination

Abdominal, genital, digital rectal, focused neurological – NAD.

Ultrasound

Bilateral grade I-II hydroureteronephrosis. Bladder wall thickness—normal, and PVR—100 mL.

Uroflometry

Uroflometry showed low flow voiding (Figure 3A, Table 1). MUPP showed low pressure-low flow voiding with no BOO (Figures 4A and B, Table 1). Absence of BOO was verified by VCUG (Figure 5).

He was advised timed voiding, tamsulosin 0.4mg OD and bethanechol 25mg tid, along with twice daily CIC to take care of post-void residue. He could not tolerate CIC and developed persistent pseudomonas bacteriuria and pyuria. Therefore, in an effort to decrease outlet resistance at EUS, we planned Botox® injection 100U in EUS.

TABLE 1: Uroflowmetry report of patient 2 one year before and immediately after injection of Botox® in EUS.

		Before Botox injection	After Botox injection
A	**Uroflowmetry**		
	Qmax (mL/s)	10	17
	Qave (mL/s)	5	10
	VV (mL)	355	567
	PVR (mL)	280	100
	cQmax	0.39	0.65
	cQave	0.20	0.38
	Voiding efficiency (%)	55.9%	85.0%
B	**MUPP**		
	pdetQmax (cm H2O)	21	32
	Qmax (mL/s)	9	14
	AG	3	4
	OCO	0.36	0.47
	Pclo at EUS (cm H2O)	−13	−14
	DAMPF	33	32
	Curve	0.12	0.05
	CHESS	A1	A1
	DCI	66	102

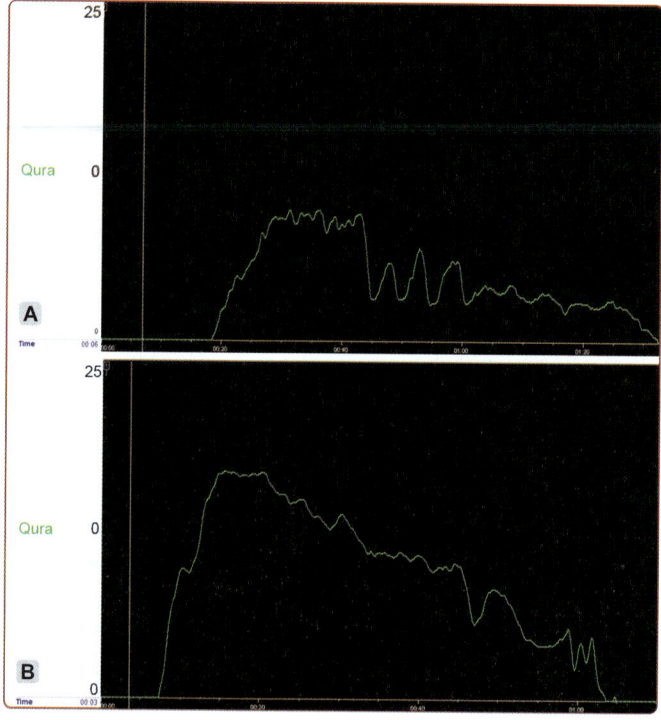

Figs 3A and B: Uroflowmetry of patient 2 (A) at presentation; (B) after Botox® injection at EUS

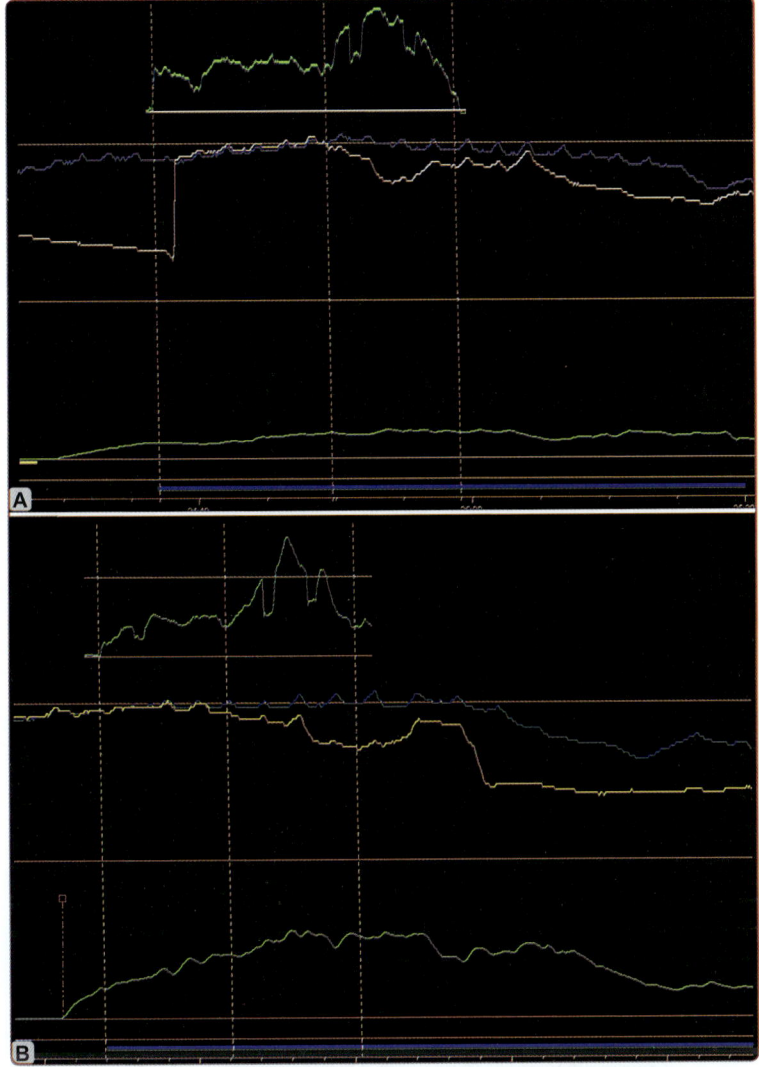

Figs 4A and B: Urethral pressure profilometry of patient 2 (A) at presentation; (B) after Botox® injection in EUS. Top tracing—resting UPP, dark blue tracing—Pves, white/yellow—Pura, bottom green tracing—Q

After the injection, he felt mild improvement of symptoms. Repeat uroflowmetry, UDS and UPP findings showed improvement in voiding efficiency (Figure 3B, Table 1). An improvement in contractility was observed; however, other urodynamic findings remained similar (Figures 4A and B, Table 1).

In view of an 'equivocal slow drainage' on nuclear urogram, we decided to perform urodynamic Whitaker test. Bilateral percutaneous nephrostomy was performed and Whitaker test was undertaken. At a variable filling rate

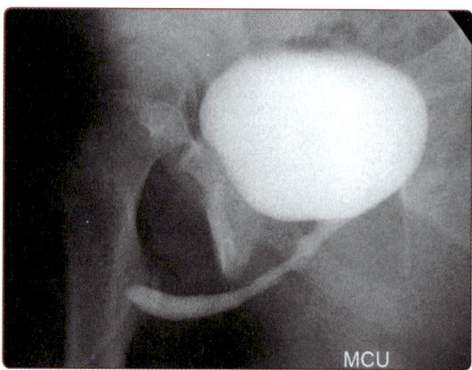

Figs 5: MCU of patient 2 showing normal bladder outlet

of 5–10 mL/min, the pressure in the right pelvicalyceal system was 8 cm H2O at initiation, which dropped to 2 cm H2O with continued filling. On the left side, initial filling pressure was 18 cm H2O which progressively, dropped to 3 cm H2O, confirming absence of obstruction on either side (Figures 6A and B).

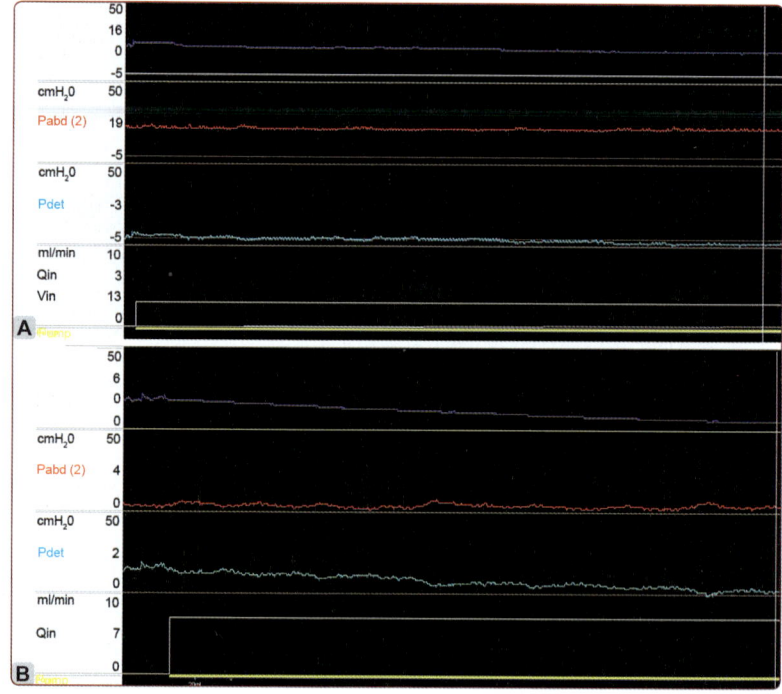

Figs 6A and B: Whitaker test of patient 2 (A) right pelvicalyceal system; (B) left pelvicalyceal system

PATIENT 3

A 52-year-old female presented with urinary urgency, frequency and difficulty in voiding for 3 years. She had three normal vaginal deliveries in the past and there was no known comorbidity. Urine culture was sterile, creatinine 1.8 mg/dL and ultrasound showed bilateral hydroureteronephrosis with thick-walled bladder and >200 mL PVR. Uroflowmetry was performed (Figure 7A) and patient catheterized for decompression. Her creatinine settled at 0.9 mg/dL and hydronephrosis resolved. Clinical examination was within normal limits for age (abdominal, pelvic, focused neurological).

Cystometry

Filling phase—Small capacity bladder (200 mL) with poor compliance (11 mL/cm H2O) and terminal detrusor overactivity. Urethral length 29 mm, MUCP—146 cm H2O.

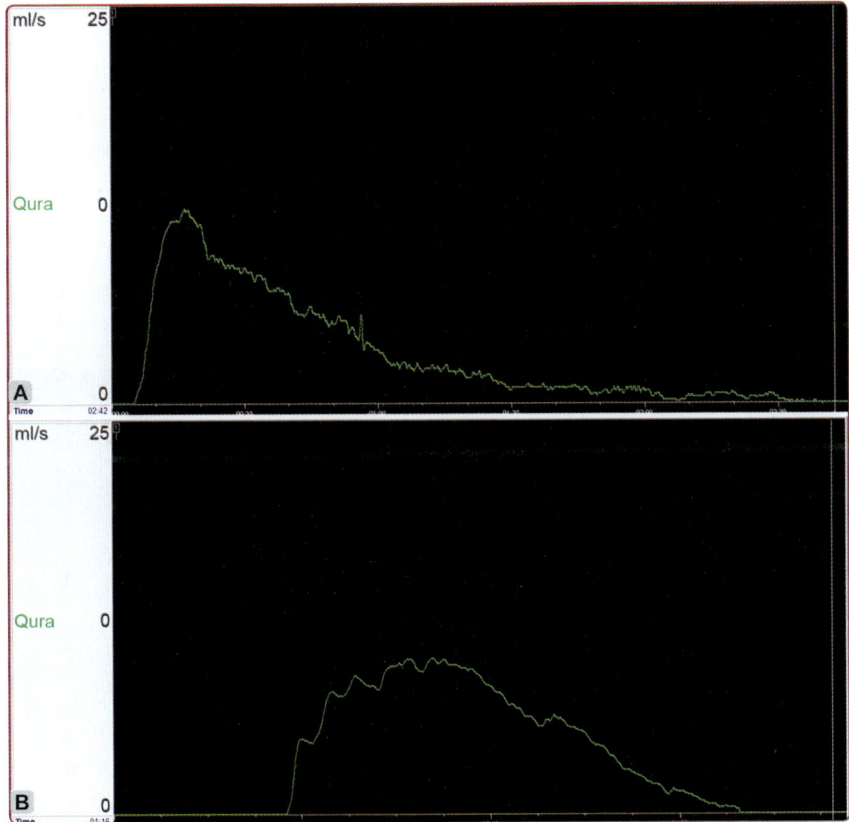

Figs 7A and B: Uroflowmetry of patient 3 (A) at presentation; (B) after treatment

Voiding phase—High pressure-low flow voiding pattern (PdetQmax 61 cm H2O, Pdetmax 74 cm H2O, Qmax 11 mL/sec). AG number-39, OCO-0.98, DAMPF-53, curve (quadratic)-0.18. CHESS plot A2. Blaivas nomogram suggested moderate obstruction.

Despite strong suspicion of BOO from these PFS parameters, MUPP revealed PClo = 0 along the entire urethra, suggestive of no BOO; this was later verified with VCUG (Figures 8A and B). The patient was taught pelvic floor exercises and prescribed tolterodine 4 mg/day, tamsulosin 0.4 mg/day. At 12 months of follow-up, she is doing well (Figure 7B).

PATIENT 4

A 23-year-old male presented with recent onset hesitancy, straining at micturition and sensation of incomplete evacuation. Clinical examination (abdominal, genital, digital rectal and focused neurological examination) was within normal limits. Uroflowmetry showed low flow pattern (Figure 9A). Ultrasound revealed a bladder diverticulum and left mild hydroureteronephrosis (Figure 10A). A urodynamic study with VCUG (for detailed depiction of diverticulum) was planned.

Cystometry

Bladder had moderate capacity (305 mL), normal compliance (35 mL/cm H2O) and phasic detrusor overactivity. Voiding phase showed a high pressure—low flow pattern (PdetQmax – 60 cm H2O; Pdetmax – 70 cm H2O Qmax – 12 mL/s; PVR – 197 mL).

AG number – 36, DAMPF – 54, OCO – 0.94, curvature – 0.17, CHESS – A2

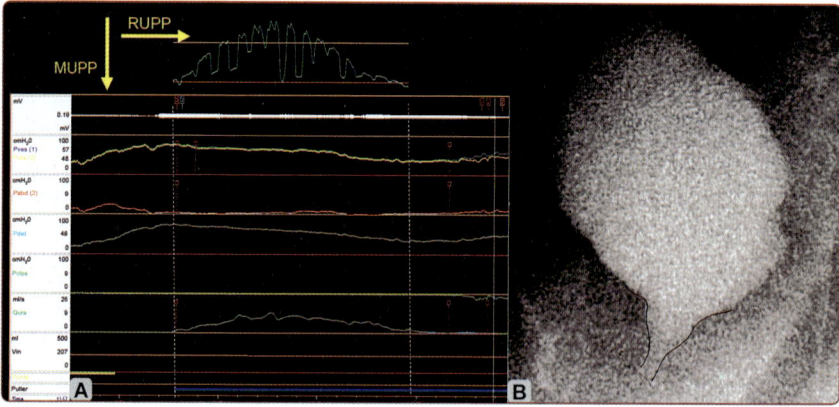

Figs 8A and B: Urodynamics of patient 3: (A) Urethral pressure profilometry showing absence of any pressure gradient between Pves and Pura indicating absence of BOO despite high pressure low flow voiding; (B) MCU verifying the UPP findings

Chapter 9 Representative Case Discussion

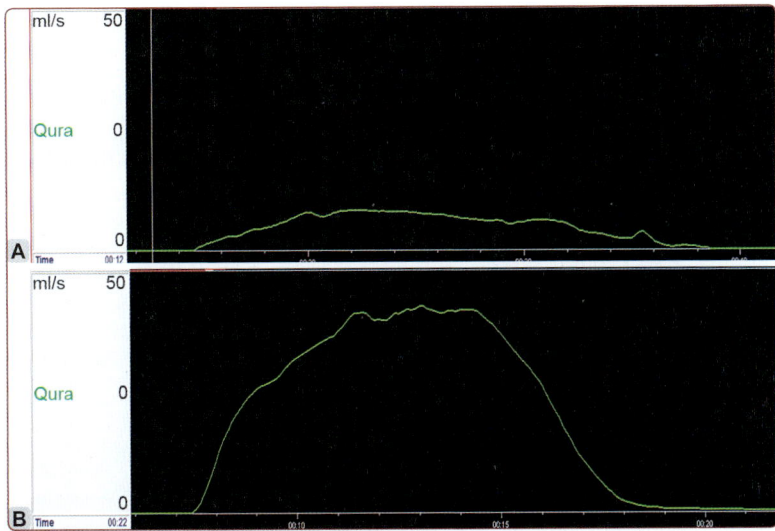

Figs 9A and B: Uroflowmetry of patient 4 (A) at presentation; (B) after surgical treatment

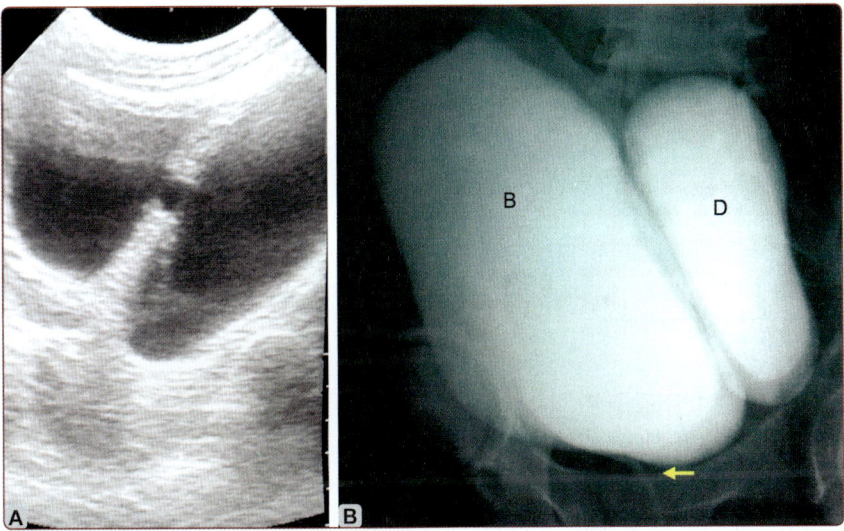

Figs 10A and B: Patient 4: (A) Ultrasound showing bladder diverticulum; (B) MCU showing diverticulum with high bladder neck—B = bladder, D = diverticulum; solid yellow arrow pointing at high bladder neck

MUPP clearly demonstrated a Pclo of −10 cm H2O starting from bladder neck suggestive of BOO (Figure 11). The question was whether to perform bladder neck incision only or with diverticulectomy. A dynamic VCUG helped in making this decision; the following pertinent findings were noted (Figure 10B):

* Neck of diverticulum ~10 mm
* Diverticulum filling concomitantly with bladder, capacity nearly 2/3rd that of bladder

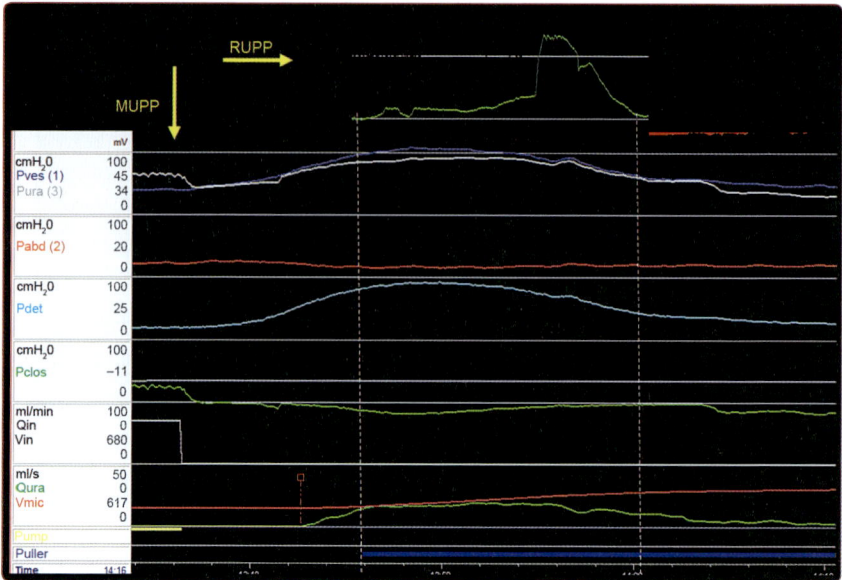

Fig. 11: Urethral pressure profilometry of patient 4. High pressure low flow pattern is observed. Pves-Pura gradient (Pclo, negative deflection in Pclo tracing) starting from bladder neck suggests bladder neck obstruction

- During voiding preferential emptying of bladder into the diverticulum; bladder neck only partially open
- Even on double voiding, diverticulum retaining significant urine.

Therefore, he underwent bladder neck incision (holmium laser) and laparoscopic diverticulectomy. He responded favorably to treatment; follow up uroflowmetry is shown in Figure 9B.

CHAPTER 10

Reporting Urodynamics

The report of urodynamics should detail each recorded component of LUT separately, in numeric as well as interpretative terms. At the end, overall impression, if possible, should be written.

Detailed components of urodynamic report:

FILLING PHASE

Bladder

1. *Sensations*—volume at first sensation, normal desire and strong desire.
   - Hyposensate—No sensations until 200 mL. Strong desire may not be reached.
   - Hypersensate—First sensation before 100 mL. The sensation persists to decrease total capacity to <250 mL.
2. *Capacity*—Numerical value.
   - Small—<200–250 mL

TABLE 1	Tabulated summary of components of a urodynamic report		
	Filling phase	*Stress phase*	*Voiding phase*
Bladder	Sensations, capacity, compliance, DO, DLPP	ALPP	Pressure, flow, volume, PVR, detrusor strength and BOO parameters
Bladder neck/prostatic urethra	Length, pressure		Vesical-urethral, Pressure-gradient, location of gradient
Sphincteric urethra	Length, pressure	Transmission ratio, ALPP	Vesical-urethral Pressure-gradient
EMG	Guarding reflex, abnormal pattern	Response with stress maneuver	Relaxation/contraction
Cystography	Outline, capacity, anatomical abnormalities	Anatomical abnormalities, status of bladder neck	Opening of bladder neck
Urethrography	Outline, anatomical abnormalities	Visibility of urethra	Status of opening, anatomical abnormalities

- Normal—300–500 mL
- Large—>500–600 mL
3. *Compliance*—Numerical value.
    - Very Low—<10–12 mL/cm H2O
    - Low—10–20 mL/cm H2O
    - Normal—20–50 mL/cm H2O
    - High—>50 mL/cm H2O
4. *Detrusor overactivity*—Presence/absence. Type-phasic or terminal.
5. *Detrusor leak-point pressure*—Abnormal >40 cm H2O.
6. *Additional comment:*

Urethra

1. *Length* of prostatic urethra/sphincteric urethra.
2. *Maximum urethral closure pressure*
    - Low (defined in females with SUI)—<20 cm H2O
    - Normal (defined in females with SUI)—>40 cm H2O
    - High (both sexes)—120–130 cm H2O
3. *Additional comment:*

EMG

Guarding reflex-present or absent/abnormal activity.

Cystography

Bladder outline/reflux/competence of bladder neck/anatomical abnormality.

STRESS PHASE

Bladder

Abdominal Leak-point pressure—numerical value.
Specify-valsalva or cough.
Any leak is abnormal.
- Low—<60 cm H2O
- Equivocal—60–90 cm H2O
- High—>90 cm H2O

Urethra

Transmission ratio—<70% suggestive of urethral hypermobility.

EMG
Cough reflex—present/absent.

Cystourethrography
Leak observed, reflux observed.

MICTURITIONAL PHASE
Bladder
1. *Voiding pattern*—(High/low) pressure—(high/low) flow, straining present/absent (straining should be avoided as far as possible).
2. PdetQmax, Pdetmax, Qmax, Qave, voided volume, PVR—numerical values.
3. *Parameters for BOO:*
   - Pmuo, AG, DAMPF, CHESS class, OCO
   - AG—<20—unobstructed; >40—obstructed; 20–40—equivocal
   - CHESS A1—unobstructed
   - OCO (defined in males)—>0.75 obstructed
   - Location of PdetQmax-Qmax point on AG nomogram, Schaefer nomogram (>grade I—obstructed), Blaivas nomogram (women).
4. *Parameters for detrusor contractility:*
   - Detrusor contractility index
     - Very weak—<50
     - Weak—50–100
     - Normal—100–150
     - Strong—>150
   - Voiding efficiency
     - Abnormal—<70–80%.

Urethra
1. Pressure gradient (Pclo) in:
   - Prostatic urethra:
     - Pclo> 5 cm H2O—yes/no
     - Location of the above from bladder neck
     - Pclomax.
   - Sphincteric urethra:
     - Pclo> 20 cm H2O—yes/no
     - Location of the above
     - Pclomax.

Cystourethrography

1. Bladder neck—obstructed/unobstructed.
2. Prostatic urethra—obstructed/unobstructed.
3. Sphincteric urethra—obstructed/unobstructed.

EMG

Status of activity—increased/decreased.

Index

Page numbers followed by 'f' and 't' indicate figures and tables respectively

A

Abdominal
  bowel diversion 23
  leak point pressure 36, 64f
  pressure 3, 23, 26, 32
  ultrasonography 19
Abnormal
  patterns of micturitional UPP 69f
  uroflow-patterns 18f
Abrams-Griffiths nomogram 44f
Acquire pressure signals from bladder 23
Actual pressure-flow curve 43f
Air-charged balloon catheter 23
Ambulatory UDS 71
Ambulatory urodynamic
  study 73f
  system 72f
Analysis of uroflowmetry graph 17f
Antegrade pressure measurement
    (APM) 75
Area under curve 37
Artifacts arising during MUPP 67f
Atmospheric pressure 32f
Average flow rate 17

B

Basic measurement transducer 16
Benign prostatic hyperplasia 20
Bilateral
  moderate hydroureteronephrosis 11
  vesicoureteral reflux 55f
Bladder
  and rectal pressures 32f
  contraction 39
  diary 9, 11f, 79
  energy 40
  filling 60
  neck
    dysfunction 20

    dyssynergia 53
    obstruction 49, 54, 80, 81, 88
    sphincter 5
  outlet
    obstruction
      compressive 18
      constrictive 18
  output relations 39, 41f
  pressure 23, 58, 62, 64
  surface 39
  urethra
    reflex 5
    pressure 23
  volume 20, 33
  wall thickness 81
Blaivas-Groutz nomogram 47f
Body mass index 20
Brainstem 6

C

Calculation of compliance 38
Calculus within ureterocele 55f
Cases of phasic detrusor overactivity 35f
Catheter
  measure hydrostatic pressure 58
  mounted microtransducers 24
  system 24
  tip transducers 58
  transducers 24
  types of 23
Cervico-dorsal spinal injuries 5
Changes in pves recording 62f
CHESS
  graph 66
  location 80
  2-dimensional plot 46f
Circumferential measurement of
    pressure 24
Collecting cylinder base of 14
Components of a urodynamic report 89t

Compression pressure 3
Compressive obstruction 18f
Compressor urethra 2f
Computer's calculation error 38
Computer-based investigation 23
Concentric needle electrode 25f
MUPP, concept of 66
Configuration of rhabdosphincter in females 2f
Connections
    circuits for UPP 60f
    frontal cortex 6
Constrictive obstruction 18f
Contraction of anal sphincter 5
Crescendo of PVES 64
Curvature of pressure-flow relation 42
Cystometric capacity 35f
Cystometry catheter 31f, 75
Cystometry filling phase 85
Cystourethrography 49, 91, 92

D

Daily
    fluid intake 11
    urine output 11
Day-time frequency 12
Deficiency of pelvic-floor 3
Delancey's hammock hypothesis 3
Description of plateau detrusor contraction pattern 47f
Design of equipment and catheters 26
Detrusor
    and fibro-elastic tissue 32
    atonia 28
    contractility index 42
    contraction
        pattern 46
        strength and volume 42, 43
    external sphincter dyssynergia 26f
    leak-point pressure 90
    overactivity index 37
    pattern 81
    pressure 26, 32, 33, 46
    sphincter dyssynergia 5, 6, 25, 54
    underactivity 18f, 19, 54
Digital rectal 8
Direct
    measure of detrusor strength 39
    visualization 36
Displacement of catheters 30f

Distal urethra 2f
Diverticulum filling 87
Double lumen 23
Double-lumen air-charged cystometry catheter 24f
Drawbacks of Whitaker test 77
Dual obstruction 81
Dynamic elastic tube 40
Dysfunctional elimination syndrome 25, 26f, 62, 63, 69, 70

E

Electrical activity of pelvic floor 25
Electrodes
    introduction 25
    setup/equipment 25
Electromechanical
    fluoroscopy- compatible urodynamic chair 16
    urodynamic chair 28
Electromyography
    electrodes 25f
    method 14
Elements of bladder wall 32
Empty rectum 27
Equivocal slow drainage 83
Etiology of obstruction 49
EUS
    dysfunction 68, 80, 81
    obstruction 80
Evaluation of clinical response 22
External sphincter
    dyssynergia 53
    zone 3f
    sphincter 25
Extravesical abdominal pressure 26
Extrinsic sphincter
    deficiency 62
    dysfunction 49

F

Fibrotic process 10
Filling
    phase compliance 33
    pressure 84
Fine double lumen cystometry catheter 29
Fixed sphincter deformity 53
Flank pain 81

Index

Flow
    pattern, type of 18
    rate 20, 33
    time 17
    volume
        nomograms 20, 21f
        index 20
Fluid infusion triple-lumen catheters 59
Fluid
    intake 9
    infused catheter 23
Fluoroscopy 36
Focused neurological 8
Fowler's syndrome 25
Function of
    bladder
        capacity 10, 12
        neck 2f, 53
    lower urinary tract 3
Functional
    external sphincter 54
    method 49
    urethra 49

G

Genital 8
Graphical representation of upper tract UDS 77f
Gravimetric (weight transducer) 14
Guarding reflex 3

H

Hand-held bladder scan 19
Hardware base unit 23
High
    osmolality contrast material 51
    power radio fluoroscopy 51
Hutch diverticulum 80
Hydrophilic guidewide 29
Hypersensate bladder 10
Hypothalamus 6

I

Infused
    volume 23, 33
    orifice 63
Injection of Botox® in EUS 82t
Integrity of
    bladder neck 53
    external sphincter 53
Intermittent
    obstruction 77
    voiding pattern 18f
Internal urethral sphincter 49
Interpretation of
    AUDS 73, 74f
    results 39, 76
Interpretation of uroflowmetry 17
Intervertebral lumbar disk 53, 54
Intrapelvic pressure IPP 76
Intraprostatic reflux 55f
Invasive concentric needle electrodes 25
Involuntary rectal activity 27f
Isovolumetric detrusor contraction 42

L

Large bladder diverticulum 55f
Leak point pressure 35, 63
Length of urethral profile 23
Liverpool nomograms for women 21f
Low flow voiding 81, 86
Lower limb reflexes 8
Lower ureteral obstruction 75
Lower urinary tract
    anatomical defect 79
    defecation 8
    dysfunction 63
    examination 8
        female-specific 8
        male-specific 8
    hematuria 7
    incontinence 7
    other symptoms 8
    pain 7
    pelvic
        examination 9
        defect 9
    severe obstructive 79
    storage symptoms 7
    symptoms history 7
    voiding symptoms 7
Luminal
    electrodes 25
    pressure 3

M

Magnetic (integral trap magnetic uroflowmeter) 14
Maximum cystometric capacity 34, 37

Maximum flow rate 17
Maximum urethral closure pressure
    (MUCP) 62, 90
MCU of patient 2 84*f*
Measure obstruction 77
Measured bladder pressure 26
Meglumine-diatrizoate solution 76
Micro-tip transducer type catheter
    systems 24
Micturitional
    phase 38, 91
    profile 80
    UPP in women patterns of 70*f*
Multichannel
    cystometry 26
    urodynamics 27
MUPP findings 80
Muscles of the pelvic floor 2

N

Natural voiding position 14
Neck of diverticulum 87
Negative diuresis renogram 77
Neural control of the lower urinary
    tract 4
Neurogenic bladder 20, 53
Neurological affliction 81
Night-time frequency 12
Non-invasive surface electrodes 25
Nonrelaxation of
    external sphincter 2*f*, 25
    sphincter 26*f*
Normal
    guarding reflex 26*f*
    micturitional urethral pressure
        profile 68*f*
    reflex response to
        cough 26*f*
        detrusor overactivity 26*f*
    silence of sphincteric 26*f*
    urine examination 11
    uroflow pattern 14*f*
    vaginal deliveries 85

O

Obstruction coefficient 44
Obstructive nephropathy 56*f*
Office UDS 71

Open-ended catheter 23
Orifice of infusion channel 59*f*
Orthotopic neobladder 40*f*
Overactive bladder 18*f*

P

Parameters for BOO 91
Parkinsonism 54
Passive urethral resistance relation
    42, 45
Peak flow rate 46
Pelvic
    cavity 3
    examination
        clitoris 9
        incontinence 9
        meatus 9
        vagina 9
    floor
        activity 26
        dysfunction 2*f*
        dysfunction 54
        exercises 86
        musculature 2
        periurethral muscles 1
        spasticity 20
        support defect schemata 9*f*
Pelvicalyceal system 77, 84
Performing the test 27
Perfusion flow study 75
Persistent obstructive symptoms 52
Phasic detrusor overactivity 86
Position of
    catheters 31
    urethra 27
Positioning of catheter 31
Posterior urethral valves 81
Postprostatectomy dysfunction 52
Postvoid residual urine 19, 27
Presence of
    catheter 27
    constant pressure 40
    high pressure 46
    sphincter spasm 29
Pressure
    Flow
        analysis 80
        relations 43
        study 23, 47*f*, 49

Index

measurement
    port 58
    principle of 23
    transducer 58
    transmission ratio 64, 65*f*
Prevailing detrusor contraction 41
Process of zeroing 32*f*
Profile length 80
Progressively increasing pelvic floor 26*f*
Projected isovolumetric contraction 42
Prophylactic antibiotic 59, 75
Prostate and external sphincter 49
Prostatic obstruction and stricture 49
Prostatic urethra 66, 67, 68, 70, 80, 89, 90, 91, 92
Proximal
    part of the urethra 3
    urethra 2*f*
Pubic symphysis 24
Pubocervical fascia 3
Pubo-urethral ligaments 3
Pubovisceralis 2
PVES orifice 59, 61, 62, 63, 66, 67, 70

R

Radiation exposure 77
Rates of urine production 77
Read and interpret uroflow data 16
Real risk of bacteremia 75
Receptacle for urine 16
Recorded parameters 37
Rectal
    catheter 31*f*
    pressure 23
Reflexes in the
    storage phase 5
    voiding phase 6
Regions of
    external sphincter 3
    cortex 6
Relaxation of
    bladder neck sphincter 5
    external sphincter 5
Renal pelvis 75, 76, 77
Reporting urodynamics 89
Representative case discussion 79
Resistance of urethral wall 61
Resting profile 80
Resting urethral pressure profile 61*f*
Retrograde urethrography 29, 52

Rhabdosphincter 1, 2, 3
Rotating disk method 14

S

Schafer nomogram 41, 44, 45*f*
Sensation symptoms of 81
Signals from
    abdomen 23
    bladder 23
    pelvic floor muscles 23
    puller 23
    pump 23
    uroflowmeter 23
Silence of
    somatic motor system 5
    sympathetic system 5
Simple
    cystometry 25
    non-invasive uroflowmetry 15
Single
    channel 25
    lumen balloon catheter 29, 30*f*
Sonesta fluoroscopic electro-mechanical motorized chair 28*f*
Sound of running water 38
Sphincter
    bradykinesia 54
    motor units 25
    spasm and pain 27
    urethra 2*f*, 89, 90, 91, 92
    urethravaginalis 2*f*
Standardized pelvic-floor prolapsed quantification system 10*f*
Sterile urine culture 26
Stimulation of parasympathetic system 5
Stop urination 80
Storage of urine 3, 4
Strength of urinary stream 13
Stress
    maneuvers 58
    phase 89
    UPP 63
    urethral pressure profilometry 36
    urinary incontinence in women 54, 63
Superior border of pubic symphysis 31
Suprasacral spinal lesions 54
Surface
    electrodes 30*f*
    EMG pattern 26*f*
    perineal electrodes 25*f*

Suspicion of BOO 86
System
   'a', PVES orifice 59
   'b' orifice 59

T

T-DOC transducers 72
Three-lumen UPP catheter 24f
Trabeculated bladder 55f
Transurethral incision of prostate 81
Triple lumen 23
Two-lumen cystometry catheter 24f

U

UDS catheters 24f
Upper tract urodynamic study 76f
Ureteropelvic junction (UPJ) 75
Ureterovesical junction (UVJ)
      obstruction 75
Urethral
   axial hypermobility (UH) 64
   bladder reflex 5, 6
   calibration 29, 52
   closure pressure 62
   hypermobility 54, 90
   part of 49, 65, 66, 67
   pressure profilometry 2f, 3f, 49, 58,
      80, 83f, 86, 88
   profile length 61
   relaxation incontinence 63
   resistance factor 46
   resistance relations 39, 41f, 66
   smooth muscle 1
   stricture 18
   vesical relation 27
Urinary
   frequency day and night 11
   leakage 63
   outflow obstruction 65
   tract infection 8
   urgency 85
      culture 85
   output 9
   production 71
Urodynamic
   lab 28

machines 58f
observation 37
patient 1 3, 80f, 86f
report 89
systems 24
Whitaker test 83
Uroflowmeter
   flow patterns 17
   measurements 16
   parts of 16f
   patient 1 79f
   patient 2 82f
   patient 3 85f
   patient 4 87f
   report 82t
   setup 15
   types of 14

V

Vaginal sponge electrode 25f
Velocities of the detrusor 18
Vesical pressure 26, 32
Vesicoureteral reflux 55f
Video urodynamic
   advantages of 54
   setup of urology service 49, 50f
Voided volume 17, 33
Voiding
   cystourethrography 49
   dysfunction 28, 66, 70, 81
   pattern 66, 69, 70, 91
   phase 5, 26f, 58, 89
Volume corrected Q 20

W

Whitaker test 75, 76, 77, 84f
Whole circuit 59

X

X-ray-compatible urodynamic chair 50

Z

Zeroing 31
Zeroing basic measurements 32